RC
489
C68
F67
2002

Forrest, Gary G.

Countertransference
in chemical

D0222341

DATE DUE

Gary G. Forrest, EdD, PhD

Countertransference in Chemical Dependency Counseling

"**D**r. Forrest has produced an important and essential book that should be required reading in all mental health graduate courses. This in-depth look at countertransference provides essential information that has not been available in a single source before. Dr. Forrest has provided a thought-provoking work that all future and current therapists could benefit from reading and applying to their professional lives."

George R. Mount, PhD
Clinical Psychologist,
Dallas, Texas

"**T**his book is a must for anyone who works with chemically dependent people. Dr. Forrest provides an in-depth look at the difficulties of not only working with those who are chemically dependent, but also, and more important, how we are impacted by these relationships. Finally, someone has recognized that we are just as affected by clients as they are by us.

The most important contributions of this book are the straightforward ways that Dr. Forrest instructs on how to handle the tasks of working with chemically dependent clients and how to maintain our health and boundaries while doing it."

Robert J. Ackerman, PhD
Director, Mid-Atlantic Addiction
Training Institute,
Indiana University
of Pennsylvania;
Author, *Perfect Daughters: Adult
Daughters of Alcoholics; Silent Sons:
A Book for and About Men;*
and *Children of Alcoholics:
A Guide for Parents, Educators,
and Therapists*

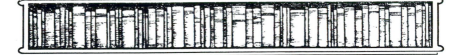

More pre-publication
REVIEWS, COMMENTARIES, EVALUATIONS . . .

"Using a style of writing that is readable, succinct, and honest, Gary Forrest has produced a remarkable book. It is the first text produced for psychotherapists and chemical dependency counselors to examine systematically and comprehensively the diverse aspects of countertransference. The text is well documented and organized; it provides a clear review of the subject that will be of value to students, active therapists and counselors, and clinical supervisors. The author provides his personal insight and promotes therapeutic relationships that use this countertransference to fuel the therapeutic process through the development of empathy, the appropriate use of clinical supervision, and the maintenance of healthy interpersonal boundaries. This book is a primer that will provide wisdom, compassion, inspiration, and comfort to those who serve the chemically dependent. I recommend it highly and without qualification."

Richard Irons, MD, FASAM
President,
Professional Renewal Center,
Lawrence, Kansas

"Dr. Forrest presents many useful insights into the very important issue of countertransference. The clinician's understanding of his or her own feelings is paramount in maximizing the therapeutic effectiveness in both the clinician and the client.

Improving diagnostic skill, constructing appropriate and workable treatment plans, and eliminating potential mistakes that can lead to treatment disasters all depend on insights discussed in this book. In addition, the subject matter could be used to construct useful in-service presentations such as treating the difficult patient and how to set realistic treatment goals.

All in all, Dr. Forrest has presented a set of insights that all who work in the field of chemical dependency will find useful. Counselor will find it helpful in improving their effectiveness, supervisors in sharpening the skills of their supervisees, and administrators in improving their staff training programs. There should be a space for this book on the shelves of all thoughtful and concerned clinicians."

Arthur P. Knauert, MD
Psychiatrist in Private Practice,
New York City

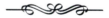

"*Countertransference in Chemical Dependency Counseling* is an enlightening analysis of an important but often ignored topic. It discusses countertransference in a way that is interesting and useful. Dr. Forrest invites us to use countertransference as a way to understand a client's needs and improve the therapeutic relationship. I expect that this text will eventually be required reading for those studying the treatment of chemical dependency."

Mike Wilbourn, PsyD
Clinical Psychologist,
The Colorado Center for Psychology,
Colorado Springs

Countertransference in Chemical Dependency Counseling

HAWORTH Addictions Treatment
F. Bruce Carruth, PhD
Senior Editor

New, Recent, and Forthcoming Titles:

Shame, Guilt and Alcoholism: Treatment Issues in Clinical Practice, Second Edition by Ronald T. Potter-Effron

Neuro-Linguistic Programming in Alcoholism Treatment edited by Chelly M. Sterman

Cocaine Solutions: Help for Cocaine Abusers and Their Families by Jennifer Rice-Licare and Katherine Delaney-McLoughlin

Preschoolers and Substance Abuse: Strategies for Prevention and Intervention by Pedro J. Lecca and Thomas D. Watts

Chemical Dependency and Antisocial Personality Disorder: Psychotherapy and Assessment Strategies by Gary G. Forrest

Substance Abuse and Physical Disability edited by Allen W. Heinemann

Addiction in Human Development: Developmental Perspectives on Addiction and Recovery by Jacqueline Wallen

Addictions Treatment for Older Adults: Evaluation of an Innovative Client-Centered Approach by Kathryn Graham, Sarah J. Saunders, Margaret C. Flower, Carol Birchmore Timney, Marilyn White-Campbell, and Anne Zeidman Pietropaolo

Group Psychotherapy with Addicted Populations: An Integration of Twelve-Step and Psychodynamic Theory, Second Edition by Philip J. Flores

Addiction Intervention: Strategies to Motivate Treatment-Seeking Behavior edited by Robert K. White and Deborah George Wright

Assessment and Treatment of the DWI Offender by Alan A. Cavaiola and Charles Wuth

Solutions for the "Treatment-Resistant" Addicted Client: Therapeutic Techniques for Engaging Challenging Clients by Nicholas A. Roes

Shame, Guild, and Alcoholism: Treatment Issues in Clinical Practice, Second Edition by Ronald T. Potter-Effron

Countertransference in Chemical Dependency Counseling by Gary G. Forrest

Countertransference in Chemical Dependency Counseling

Gary G. Forrest, EdD, PhD

The Haworth Press®
New York • London • Oxford

The Haworth Press, Inc., 10 Alice Street, Binghamton, NY 13904-1580

Cover design by Anastasia Litwak.

Library of Congress Cataloging-in-Publication Data

Forrest, Gary G.
    Countertransference in chemical dependency counseling / Gary G. Forrest
        p. cm.
    Includes bibliographical references and index.
    ISBN 0-7890-1523-4 (hard : alk. paper)—ISBN 0-7890-1524-2 (soft : alk. paper)
    1. Countertransference (Psychology) 2. Narcotic addicts—Counseling of. 3. Alcoholics—Counseling of. I. Title.

RC489.C68 F67 2001
616.86'0651—dc21

2001016624

To my family, and especially my mother,
Florence "Flossie" Forrest-Summy,
extended family, friends, and colleagues;
my patients over the past thirty years;
and to Bruce A. Montoya and Matthew R. Groves,
the guardians of my soul from November 1998
through February 2000

ABOUT THE AUTHOR

Gary G. Forrest, EdD, PhD, is a licensed clinical psychologist in full-time independent practice in Colorado Springs, Colorado. He has been involved in the treatment of alcoholics, substance abusers, and their families for over twenty-five years. A nationally recognized speaker and educator, he is Executive Director of Psychotherapy Associates, PC, and the Institute for Addictive Behavioral Change in Colorado Springs. Dr. Forrest is also Executive Director of the International Academy of Behavioral Medicine, Counseling, and Psychotherapy as well as the author of *Chemical Dependency and Antisocial Personality Disorder: Psychotherapy and Assessment Strategies* (Haworth, 1994). He has authored numerous textbooks and professional publications.

CONTENTS

Foreword

Very few of us have escaped the pervasive impacts that addiction wreaks on individuals and their families. None of us have escaped the attitudes and perceptions our culture holds for the alcoholic and drug addict. As therapists and counselors, all of us have been affected, for better or worse, by the behaviors of our addicted clients. Thus, our countertransferential responses—the attitudes, values, beliefs, and expectations we bring from our history into the therapy office and unconsciously project onto the client—are of significant importance in our work with chemically dependent people.

However, surprisingly little scientific study has been devoted to the topic of countertransferential dynamics with chemically dependent patients. Dr. Forrest offers us a comprehensive, dynamic, and well-researched look at how countertransference affects counseling and psychotherapy with addicts and their families. He challenges readers to examine their own needs, psychosocial history, values, ethics, and professional responsibilities. His insights into the nature of countertransference illuminate an often deeply buried and superficially addressed topic.

Chemically dependent patients have a unique ability to provoke our own history. In early recovery, they excite our rescue fantasies by improving rapidly. Similarly, their relapses have the potential to activate our sense of impotence. We shift from therapist to parent, offering well-intentioned advice and admonishments. The addicted client activates our past experience with addicted people in our own lives. Also, of course, in this field, where so many of the care providers are recovering addicts themselves, a counselor's experience of his or her own recovery cannot help but affect how the counselor relates to the recovery needs of the client.

As Dr. Forrest aptly points out, countertransference is inherently neither good nor bad, neither right nor wrong; it is just part of the mix that is the intimate, therapeutic contact between two people. It does, however, need to be recognized and addressed as such. In this era of "mechanized therapy," where individuals are pushed through the change process with emphasis on time and dollar constraints, where therapists and counselors get less and less true clinical supervision, where continuing education is provided in groups numbering in the hundreds, and where personal therapy and growth opportunities for care providers are not supported, countertransferential dynamics remain unrecognized and unaddressed in the therapeutic mix. In the words of twelve-step wisdom, we "keep doing what we've always done and get what we've always gotten."

Countertransference in Chemical Dependency Counseling is a groundbreaking book in confronting therapist and counselor reactions to the chemically dependent patient. I hope you will find it as illuminating as I have.

Bruce Carruth, PhD, LCSW
Senior Editor, Addictions Treatment
The Haworth Press Book Series

Acknowledgments

Many individuals contributed to this book. I continue to learn a great deal from my clients, and in the context of this work, they have made me more aware of my own countertransference reactions and how these reactions influence and affect our relationships and functioning. Our clients, supervisors and educators, colleagues, families, and significant others remain our lifelong teachers! My ongoing collegial relationships with L. E. Wellman, EdD; Dennis Caldwell, MD; Barb Martin, LCSW; and Mike Wilbourn, PsyD, have made it easier to understand and write about countertransference in chemical dependency counseling. My typist, Mary DeShong, is really responsible for bringing this book to fruition. She typed the original draft of this manuscript and then, after some eighteen months, retyped the manuscript, placed it on my office desk one day, and commented, "I think it's time for us to finish this book." Again, thanks to Mary! Finally, as always, my family and extended family have been supportive and encouraging—Sandra, Sarah, Allison, Floss, Lindy, Victor and Ellen, and Victor—and to everyone else, a loving thanks!

When drunk, I made them pay and pay and pay and pay.

F. Scott Fitzgerald

Is it any wonder that these clients [addicts and substance abusers] provoke such a wide range of intense emotional reactions and responses in chemical dependency counselors and other health service providers?

Gary G. Forrest

They're always very difficult to work with [chemically dependent persons] . . . but women are especially difficult for me. . . . I'm always reminded of myself, and the worst of me. For a long time, I couldn't work with alcoholic women.

Carrie W., MA, CAC III
Recovering Chemical
Dependency Counselor

Chapter 1

Introduction

Chemically dependent and substance-abusing clients stir a multiplicity of feelings, thoughts, and reactions in counselors and other health service providers with whom they become involved. Counselors "like" some clients while they may dislike others. Counselors find it difficult to communicate effectively with some clients, may fear certain clients, find it difficult to establish a working and productive therapeutic alliance with some, distrust others, and find themselves being abused or verbally attacked by a few of their chemically dependent clients. They may consciously respect, love, or even feel physically attracted to some of their substance-abusing clients.

Alcoholics and substance abusers are consistently difficult to treat, and notoriously disliked or avoided by counselors, psychologists, physicians, and other helping professionals (Bratter and Forrest, 1985; Weiss, 1994; Forrest, 1997b, 1998a, 2001). However, there have always been a few health providers who have chosen to work with this clinical population. Many of these clinicians also report both personal satisfaction and successful client treatment outcomes as a result of this career choice. Over the past decade, chemical dependency counseling and addictions treatment has evolved into a true behavioral health career and profession, and this "new profession" consistently attracts individuals from all health care specialty areas.

Many economic, social, political, and psychological factors have contributed to the evolution and development of chemical dependency treatment alternatives in the United States and throughout the world. Certainly, a major variable in this process has been the demand and need for treatment services for a growing population of substance abusers and chemically dependent persons in any given population or society. Furthermore, these individuals impact all of our lives in myriad ways, and they end up costing the American collective millions of dollars each day. The American and international drug war has been fought and continually lost for decades. In America, we simply cannot build enough prisons, correctional facilities, or treatment programs to treat and/or incarcerate our exploding offender population, which includes hundreds of thousands of substance abusers and chemically dependent persons (Forrest and Gordon, 1990; Forrest, 2000). Moreover, we cannot spend enough money or build these facilities fast enough to warehouse this ever-growing segment of American society.

The media have recently played a major role in the process of confronting and breaking down our collective denial about drug addiction and substance abuse in America and elsewhere in the world. Every day we are confronted with the realities of addicted police officers, mayors, doctors, housewives, professional athletes, famous movie stars and media figures, lawyers, corporate executives, teens, educators, airline pilots, clergy, and so forth. We see these people on television. We read about them, know them, hear about them on the radio, and live with them. Indeed, we know them well because they are us—we are beginning to understand that substance abuse and chemical dependency are illnesses, disorders, or diseases that can and do affect virtually all Americans.

Is it any wonder that as individuals, as well as collectively, we are ambivalent about the various issues associated with chemical dependency and substance abuse in the United States? We generally want the drug dealers locked up, but not our substance-abusing sons or daughters, spouses, or parents. We employ Employee Assistance Program (EAP) specialists to identify drug abusers in the workplace, but we are uncomfortable about requiring our chief executive officers (CEOs) to take random urinalysis tests. Alcohol is a legal drug, but heroin, marijuana, and methamphetamine are illegal drugs. Communities are shaken when the local priest, school superintendent, or physician enters a chemical dependency treatment program or is arrested for driving under the influence (DUI). Individuals who manifest a major depressive disorder or perhaps schizophrenia have a bona fide mental illness and are deserving of real or quality medical and psychiatric care. How about substance abusers and addicts? Yet, the reality remains. There are far more alcoholics, substance abusers, and chemically dependent persons in any general or random population of people than there are schizophrenics, depressives, or persons with cancer, leukemia, heart disease, multiple sclerosis, cystic fibrosis, diabetes, or Alzheimer's disease.

Perhaps our generalized ambivalence about chemical dependency is largely related to the matter of choice. Most people believe that alcoholics choose to drink or remain abstinent and are, thus, responsible for their purported disease or illness. Likewise, people who smoke cigarettes or marijuana, inject narcotics intravenously, become addicted to prescription medications, or abuse other psychoactive substances are generally responsible for the various consequences of their drug-taking and drug-related behaviors. Although these beliefs and ideologies remain grist for debate and discussion, our ambivalence about the various issues associated with chemical dependency and substance abuse can be traced to another source: *countertransference.*

Countertransference is an ever-present reality that impacts the lives and social interactions (La Roche, 1999) of all individuals. However, this text examines the various roles of countertransference in the explicit realm of chemical dependency counseling. Many chemical dependency counselors are generally unfamiliar with the concept of countertransference, and this topic has remained poorly understood in the mental health and behavioral health fields. Chemical dependency counselors and mental health workers are far more familiar with the concept of transference, and, indeed, clinicians have long blamed their treatment failures on the transference reactions of their clients. The author's opinion is that countertransference contributes to treatment outcome failures and a plethora of other relational difficulties that consistently occur within the context of chemical dependency counseling, and in virtually all psychotherapy or counseling relationships.

Countertransference (1) reflects the unconscious and neurotic conflicts of the counselor or therapist, as well as his or her total being; (2) is usually related to the client's transference, personality, and behavior; (3) is an inevitable and desirable component of the

counseling or psychotherapy relationship; (4) can potentially foster growth, education, and change upon the part of the counselor
and client as well as within the context of the helping relationship;
and (5) may destructively impact the counselor, client, and therapeutic relationship.

Several definitions and historical perspectives of countertransference are provided in Chapter 2. Countertransference in the specific realm of chemical dependency counseling is examined in
Chapter 3. Countertransference distortion is defined and the sources
of countertransference distortion in chemical dependency counseling are elucidated in Chapter 4. Techniques and strategies for
resolving and managing countertransference distortion in chemical
dependency counseling are provided in Chapter 5. The constructive and therapeutic dimensions of countertransference in chemical dependency counseling are discussed in Chapter 6. Chapter 7
includes a general discussion of contemporary and future issues
related to countertransference in chemical dependency counseling
and psychotherapy: ethics, gender, and multicultural realities; managed care; and client comorbidity/dual diagnosis. The final chapter
summarizes the material presented in earlier chapters and reveals
some of the author's recent conflictual countertransference reactions.

This book is the first to comprehensively address the topic of
countertransference in chemical dependency counseling. All chemical dependency counselors, psychologists, psychiatrists, social
workers, and other health service providers who work with substance abusers and chemically dependent persons will find this
book to be very informative and pragmatically useful in their treatment relationships with this clinical population.

Dr. Shaffer (1994) has noted that chemical dependency and
mental health treatment providers have traditionally associated
treatment failures or stalemates with client traits. I agree with
Shaffer's position that treatment failures come from provider
countertransference and poor treatment client matches. This book
was written to help chemical dependency counselors and other substance abuse treatment personnel become more effective in their
treatment relationships by better understanding, resolving and

managing, and constructively utilizing countertransference phenomena.

As there has always been a dearth of basic and applied research dealing with countertransference and the therapist's emotional reactions to substance abusers (Levin, 1991; Najavits et al., 1995; Forrest, 1997b; Carruth, 2000), I also hope that the present text is heuristic in addition to enhancing the general therapeutic armamentarium of all chemical dependency counselors and substance abuse treatment personnel.

Chapter 2

Countertransference: Historical Perspectives and Definitions

INTRODUCTION

The concept of countertransference has been discussed and examined in the psychotherapy and behavioral science literature for nearly one hundred years. Countertransference is a psychoanalytic concept, and psychoanalytically oriented psychotherapists continue to elucidate the various aspects of this concept (Slakter, 1987; Shaffer, 1994; Hahn, 2000). During the past three decades, several "schools" of counseling and psychotherapy have incorporated various aspects of the countertransference concept. Thus, countertransference phenomena may be discussed within the context of behavioral science literature specific to any and/or all approaches to counseling and psychotherapy.

The various relational, sexual, political, financial, familial and marital, legal, societal, and emotional or psychological reactions that were associated with the President Clinton–Monica Lewinsky relationship can be viewed as countertransference phenomena. The reality of countertransference stirred a variety of intense feelings, thoughts, and reactions in most Americans of 1998 and 1999 as they experienced the unfolding of the Clinton-Lewinsky relationship in the news media on a daily basis. The president of the United States is clearly akin to a counselor or physician in his professional roles as leader, father figure, international role model, helper and healer, protector, boss or employer, and so forth. Monica Lewinsky was also akin to a client or patient in her relationship to and with President Clinton.

Regardless of the specifics of the Clinton-Lewinsky relationship, it is the author's belief that both Mr. Clinton and Ms. Lewinsky experienced many or all of the various feelings, cognitions, and reactions that are discussed throughout the course of this text. Furthermore, Mr. Clinton and Ms. Lewinsky will, in all probability, be dealing with these countertransference issues for the remainder of their lives.

Chemical dependency counseling is a new and emerging profession within the behavioral science field (Bratter and Forrest, 1985; Forrest, 1992, 1997b, 2000, 2001). The concept of countertransference has received very little attention in the recently evolving substance abuse and chemical dependency treatment literature. This chapter examines the history of the countertransference concept and historic as well as current definitions of countertransference. The definitional parameters of countertransference presented in this chapter will help the reader understand and more fully appreciate the complex countertransference-oriented issues addressed in subsequent chapters.

HISTORY AND DEFINITIONS

Freud (1961/1910) initially discussed the concept of countertransference in *Future Prospects for Psycho-Analytic Therapy*. He wrote:

> We have become aware of the "counter-transference" [Gegen-ubertragung] which arises in [the physician] as a result of the unconscious feelings and we are almost inclined to insist that he shall recognize this counter-transference in himself and overcome it. (pp. 141-142)

Freud (1961/1912) also described countertransference as the analyst's use of his own unconscious to understand the patient's unconscious:

> To put it into a formula: The analyst must turn his own unconscious like a receptive organ toward the transmitting unconscious of the patient. He must adjust himself to the patient as

a telephone receiver is adjusted to the transmitting microphone. (p. 111)

It should be noted that Freud actually wrote very little about countertransference. However, it is clear that Freud used countertransference to refer to the analyst's blind spots that were obstacles to analysis. Countertransference in the analyst was equated with resistance in the patient.

Many Freudian psychoanalysts as well as neo-Freudian and contemporary analysts have written about countertransference. Although Freud's early successors generally ignored the topic of countertransference, Ferenczi (1950/1919) defined "objective countertransference" as "the analyst's emotional reactions to the real personality of the patient" (p. 104). He noted that the doctor "is always a human being" and went so far as to suggest that, in certain circumstances, the analyst should reveal his (or her) feelings and even mistakes to the patient. Ferenczi recognized that (negative) countertransference reflects the analyst's reactions to the patient's transference in combination with the analyst's unresolved oedipal conflicts.

Stern (1924), Deutsch (1953/1926), Glover (1927), Reich (1945/1933), Fleiss (1942), Fromm-Reichmann (1950), Menninger and Holzman (1958), and several other early analysts provided definitions of countertransference. These definitions generally emphasized that countertransference reactions

1. reflect the unconscious neurotic conflicts of the analyst;
2. are related to the patient's transference, personality, and behavior;
3. are an inevitable and even desirable component of the process of psychoanalytic treatment;
4. can foster growth and enhanced self-awareness upon the part of the analyst and the patient; and
5. can destructively impact the patient and the analyst as well as impede the psychoanalytic process.

It is apparent that evolving definitions of countertransference take into account the "real person" dimensions of the analyst and openly acknowledge that the patient can have a profound effect upon the analyst. Furthermore, psychoanalysis and other psychotherapies involve intimate human relationships. Whereas Freud and the early Freudians denied the existence of strong feelings in the analyst, Winnicott (1949) and subsequent psychoanalytic authors openly acknowledge that *all* analysts have intense feelings toward their patients, they are entitled to these feelings, and the affective reactions of the analyst should be a part of the treatment process. Thus, Gitelson (1952) defines countertransference as "the analyst's reactions to the patient's transference, to the material the patient brings in, and to the patient's response to him as a person" (p. 3). The patient's perceptions, responses, feelings, and intuitive understanding of the analyst clearly impact the analyst and the psychoanalytic relationship.

Heimann (1950) extended the definition of countertransference to include *all* of the analyst's feelings toward the patient. She believed that countertransference can be "an instrument of research into the patient's unconscious" and argued that it is a tool for understanding the patient as well as the analyst. The revisionistic viewpoints of Heimann and Winnicott on countertransference facilitated further investigations of the topic.

During the late 1950s through the 1970s, several psychoanalytic authors examined the interactional nature of countertransference. Tower (1956), Searles (1958, 1975), Kernberg (1965, 1975), Bleger (1967), Greenson (1971), Langs (1978), Giovacchini (1979), and Gill (1979) focus upon different dimensions of the interactive and relational nature of countertransference. For example, Searles (1975) believes that once the patient begins to understand some of the analyst's unconscious conflicts, the patient will frequently attempt to cure the analyst by acting as the analyst's analyst. Langs (1978) indicated that countertransference can be understood only within the context of a "bipersonal field." According to Langs:

> Having an office separate from his home, always starting and ending a session on time, never taking notes or answering the telephone during a session, never eating in the patient's presence, and keeping his private life entirely private . . . when the

analyst breaks any of these rules, he is demonstrating count-ertransference. And the more often he breaks them, the more difficulty he will have in understanding his reasons for doing so and hence in conducting a successful analysis. (p. 33)

Giovacchini (1979), McDougall (1979), and Gill (1979) explore the differences in countertransference reactions associated with treating psychotics and schizophrenics rather than neurotics. These authors point out that many clinicians experience extreme anxiety and discomfort in their treatment relationships with psychotics. Giovacchini (1979) indicates that the patient helps reveal to the analyst the analyst's countertransference reactions; thus, the patient teaches the analyst how to treat him or her. He states that "we treat the untreatable in order to receive treatment ourselves" (p. 18). McDougall (1979) notes that countertransference feelings of self-doubt and resentment can create "inbuilt hesitance" in the analyst that makes it difficult for the analyst to hear what the patient is communicating. The analyst's authoritarianism may be associated with fear and anxiety about identifying with the patient.

Many contemporary psychoanalysts contend that countertransference is not necessarily harmful or destructive to the analytic process. Brenner (1977) states:

Countertransference is ubiquitous and inescapable, just as is transference. Countertransference is the transference of the analyst in an analytic situation. Becoming an analyst, practicing analysis, necessarily involves, for each individual analyst, derivatives of that analyst's childhood conflicts.There is nothing pathological or neurotic in this. It is, in fact, as inevitable for the profession of analysis as it is for the choice and practice of any other vocation. Instances of countertransference which interfere with analysis are examples of pathological or neurotic compromise formation. (p. 44)

Searles (1987) utilizes a definition of countertransference provided by the American Psychoanalytic Association: "Countertransference refers to the attitudes and feelings, only partly conscious, of the analyst toward the patient" (p. 29). He notes that "countertransference gives one one's most reliable approach to the understanding of patients of whatever diagnosis" (p. 131). He also indicates that the analyst may introject some of the patient's psychopathology and even experience (countertransference psychosis) problems differentiating between self and the patient. Searles (1965) emphasizes that any diagnostic formulation should begin with studying the interviewer's emotional reactions in the interaction between the patient and the interviewer.

As Blum (1987) points out, countertransference is not a term that is easily defined. Classic definitions of countertransference focus upon impediments and interferences with the analyst's neutrality, empathy, and interpretations in the analytic process. Blum (1987) astutely notes that "analysis is a very complex intimate profession with many occupational hazards." Attempts to openly discuss countertransference issues are frequently avoided by the psychoanalytic community. He also indicates that

> (1) analysts are vulnerable to all human frailties, to conflict and regression, (2) the analyst may have neurotic reactions to any aspect of the patient and not only to the transference, (3) the analyst's personal life ("agenda") may be associated with his vulnerability to countertransference reactions and/or the extension of his personal problems with his professional work, (4) countertransference is often related both to the specific features of the patient's transference and to the analyst's character pathology, (5) the chronically angry analyst will be prone to acute and specific negative countertransference, (6) too much therapeutic zeal and rescue fantasies, loss of therapeutic interest and concern with boredom, or subtle devaluation of the patient's efforts at mastery, and silence or speech changes (pitch, pressure, syntax) can be indicators of countertransference, and (7) countertransference reactions to termination are common. (pp. 88-93)

Blum (1987) defines analytic countertransference as a "counterreaction to the patient's transference which is unconscious and indicative of the analyst's own unresolved intrapsychic conflicts" (p. 90). He seems generally to accept Freud's (1961/1910) observation that no psychoanalyst goes further than his (or her) own complexes and internal resistances permit.

Several practical symptoms of countertransference are provided by Savage (1987). These include

1. analyzing in the patient what really exists in oneself,
2. failing to see in the patient what one does not want to see in oneself, and
3. using the patient to obtain substitute gratification.

This author also notes that countertransference is an anxiety-provoking topic within the psychoanalytic community, in part, because it threatens the medical code, which places all of the disease in the patient.

Recurrent thoughts about the patient, a repetitive or compulsive need to talk about the patient, dreaming about the patient, and even matters pertaining to billing and making appointment arrangements may be indicators of countertransference. Slakter (1987) correctly indicates that

> if the therapist is seduced—that is, if he has an affair with the patient—then he is responding not just to reality but also to the countertransference. In doing so, he is creating a new reality situation, one that is bound to destroy the treatment. (pp. 223-224)

He also believes that gender issues, character traits, liking, reality factors, personality and culture, and the patient's expectations can be related to countertransference. Although there is no singular "right or wrong" method for dealing with fees, Slakter (1987) states that "sliding scales are fertile breeding ground for transference and countertransference." Refusal to pay treatment fees and similar patient tactics associated with the monetary nature of the therapeutic relationship predictably result in countertransference reactions.

Tansey and Burke (1989) broadly define countertransference as

> [t]he therapist's total response to the patient, both conscious and unconscious. This "total response" includes all the

thoughts and feelings that the therapist experiences in reaction to the therapeutic interaction whether they are considered to be "real" or "neurotically distorted." (p. 41)

These authors view transference as an umbrella term that encompasses the concepts of projective identification, introjective identification, and empathy. They note that Reik (1948) stated, "the psychoanalyst is a human being like any other and not a god. There is nothing superhuman about him" (p. 154). In this regard, Tansey and Burke (1989) indicate that the therapist's strong emotional responses to the patient are not necessarily indicative of emotional problems in the therapist.

It has been noted (Tansey and Burke, 1989) that "all therapists work well with certain types of patients and less, or even poorly, with others" (p. 75). These authors believe that early in treatment, it is often the gross characteristics of the patient that elicit disruptions in the "mental set" of the therapist. They also refer to Sullivan's (1953) concepts of "difficulties in living" and "we are all much more simply human than otherwise," note Freud's personal countertransference distortions in his analysis of the Wolfman, and purport that attempting to make sense of countertransference material is inescapably inferential and hermeneutical.

Levin (1991) indicates that countertransference

in the broad sense tells us something about ourselves and something about the patient. Our feelings while working with patients provide us with data about our own mental processes and unresolved conflicts, and with vital data about patients' mental processes and their effects on people; they are a unique source of information, providing us with insights not otherwise available. (p. 267)

Levin (1991) also believes that countertransference is always present in the counseling relationship and that it is essential for counselors to be aware of countertransference feelings; "otherwise, they will be acted out, to the detriment of the treatment" (p. 268).

Weiss (1994) points out that contemporary definitions of countertransference include thoughts and feelings of the psychotherapist evoked by the patient's dynamics. She also astutely observes that countertransferential feelings emerge in various forms between patients and health service providers other than psychotherapists.

Shaffer (1994) examines the dynamics of denial, ambivalence, and countertransferential hate within the context of psychotherapy relations with chemically dependent persons. In this brilliant and provocative chapter, Shaffer notes that clinicians need to "identify their real feelings—which may offer little to the conduct of psychotherapy—and distinguish these from countertransference, which can be extremely helpful" (p. 428). He examines the various sources of countertransferential hate in depth.

Very recent psychoanalytically and dynamically oriented authors (Hahn, 2000; Dalenberg, 2000) examine the impact of countertransference upon the process and outcome of psychotherapy relationships with special patient subpopulations.

Counseling and substance abuse literature currently (Forrest, 1998a, 2000; Culbreth and Borders, 1999; Carruth, 2000; Hansen, 2000) relies less upon the use of the countertransference construct to understand and describe the various relational aspects between the counselor and chemically dependent client. Countertransference-oriented dynamics pertaining to the counseling relationship are often examined within such contexts as supervisory relationships between recovering and nonrecovering substance abuse counselors (Culbreth and Borders, 1999), difficult clients (Carruth, 2000), and special or multicultural populations (Marotta and Asner, 1999; Britton, Cimini, and Rak, 1999; Aspy et al., 2000; Forrest, 2000). Nonetheless, it is very apparent that all of these "new" areas of counselor or therapist training, supervision and education, clinical practice, and even research investigation pertain to countertransference.

SUMMARY

Countertransference was originally a Freudian psychoanalytic concept (Freud, 1961/1910). In general, countertransference refers to the analyst's feelings and reactions to the patient. The early Freudian analysts (Stern, 1924; Fleiss, 1942; Fromm-Reichmann, 1950) emphasized that (1) countertransference should ideally be eliminated from the therapeutic relationship, and (2) counter-transference reactions reflect the unconscious neurotic conflicts of the analyst. Contemporary analysts (Slakter, 1987; Tansey and Burke, 1989; Hahn, 2000) view countertransference as an inevitable and even desirable aspect of psychoanalysis and psychoanalytically oriented psychotherapy. Dalenberg (2000) has recently explored countertransference within the specific realm of trauma treatment.

Analysts and psychotherapists (Navajavits et al., 1995) have generally been reluctant to examine the effects of countertransference upon the process and outcome of psychotherapy. This is understandable, as countertransference is a complex, multifaceted, and ubiquitous concept that is not easily defined. Countertransference is the transference of the therapist within the context of the therapeutic relationship.

Countertransference reflects the imperfect human qualities and characteristics of the psychotherapist. Viewed from this perspective, countertransference can contribute to the manifestation of various problems in the treatment relationship as well as enhance the therapeutic process or the outcome of psychotherapy. Indeed, countertransference colors, affects, and shapes, for better or worse (Forrest, 1998a, 1999, 2000; Britton, Cimini, and Rak, 1999; Carruth, 2000), the various dimensions of the process and outcome of psychotherapy as well as psychoanalysis.

From a broader perspective, it was noted at the beginning of the chapter that a wide variety of countertransference phenomena were associated with the President Clinton–Monica Lewinsky relationship. Clearly, countertransference can reflect the imperfect qualities of all people and can contribute to the development of a variety of problems and conflicts in all human relationships. The "for better or worse" impact of countertransference is clearly not limited to the professional therapeutic or counseling relationship.

Chapter 3

Countertransference and the Process of Chemical Dependency Counseling

INTRODUCTION

As noted in the introduction to Chapter 1, chemical dependency counseling is a new and emergent career field within the mental health or behavioral science professions. Chemical dependency counselors have traditionally received very little formal academic training in the areas of mental health, psychology, family therapy, behavioral medicine and psychiatry, or social work. Many chemical dependency counselors have entered this profession as a result of the personal experience of being a client or patient and via the process of recovery. These individuals tend to be unfamiliar with the concept of countertransference and other basic psychological terms and constructs.

The chemical dependency counseling profession is a growing, changing, and evolving career field. As such, chemical dependency counselors are now certified and must complete various continuing education and training requirements, and increasing numbers of these individuals complete undergraduate and graduate training in counseling, psychology, social work, family therapy, and the behavioral science disciplines. Professionally trained, experienced, and supervised chemical dependency counselors are becoming increasingly cognizant of the impact of countertransference upon the process and outcome of chemical dependency counseling and treatment (Forrest, 1997b).

This chapter includes an examination of countertransference in chemical dependency counseling. Countertransference is a central and influential component in all psychotherapy and counseling relationships with substance abusers and chemically dependent patients.

COUNTERTRANSFERENCE DYNAMICS AND REACTIONS IN CHEMICAL DEPENDENCY COUNSELING

There is a marked dearth of information pertaining to countertransference in the chemical dependency counseling and treatment literature. However, Forrest (1998a, 1999) defined countertransference within the context of intensive alcoholism psychotherapy as follows:

> The therapist's inappropriate and neurotic reactions to the patient and the psychotherapy relationship. The psychotherapeutic process sometimes exacerbates the psychotherapist's unresolved infantile and familial conflicts. Thus, the therapist begins to interact neurotically with the patient as he or she did with early-life significant others. Countertransference reactions can result in psychonoxious psychotherapy. (1997b, p. 84)

Forrest (1997b) also notes that (1) countertransference conflicts can be related to the unconscious and preconscious behaviors and beliefs that the therapist models in the psychotherapeutic relationship, and (2) therapist countertransference distortions are frequently manifestations of overdetermined "rescuing" during the early stages of intensive alcoholism psychotherapy.

Forrest (1979) has also related countertransference to the processes of suicidal acting out and successful suicide attempts in psychotherapy with alcoholics and chemically dependent patients. This author (Forrest, 1992) states:

> A basic psychodynamic consideration in therapeutic work with alcoholic patients, as with other patients, has to do with our countertransference distortion related to rescuing or saving the patient. The alcoholic entering treatment is often depressed, overwhelmed, and literally "begging for help." As such, the alcoholic sets the therapist up for assuming a rescu-

ing position . . . as a result, such counselors and therapists tend to construct highly dependent relationships with their patients in which superficial sobriety and behavioral change depend upon the on-going rescuing transactions of the therapist. Ultimately, such a psychotherapy alliance suffers an irreversible impasse. In fact, the alcoholic patient may be killed by this form of on-going transaction. (pp. 28-29)

Psychonoxious confrontation styles or transactions (Forrest, 1992, 1999) evolve from the countertransference distortions of the therapist. Anger, rejection, and patient dislike form the nuclear core of the therapist's pathologic confrontations. The catagogic or neurotic trends (countertransference) of the psychotherapist are exacerbated by the iconoclastic attitudes and pathologic confrontational style of the chemically dependent client. Iatrogenic confrontation strategies (Forrest, 1992) tend to evolve from the therapist's feelings of frustration, anger, and, at times, poorly controlled rage.

Forrest (1992, 1997b, 1998a) indicates that the interpersonal style of the alcoholic tends to generate countertransference distortion. As countertransference factors become increasingly significant and operational within the context of an intensive chemical dependency counseling relationship, the therapist may unwittingly sabotage the therapeutic alliance vis-à-vis active movement into the role of a primary persecutor (Forrest, 1979).

It should also be noted that several clinicians (Forrest, 1978, 1991, 1994; Wegscheider, 1981; Zimberg, 1982; Bratter and Forrest, 1985; Wallace, 1985; Gorski and Miller, 1986; Gorski, 1992; Weiss, 1994; Culbreth and Borders, 1999; Carruth, 2000) have indicated that chemically dependent patients can be very difficult to treat. These authors note that chemically dependent patients tend to evoke intense and personally disturbing emotions in the therapist. Although these clinicians have not usually employed the concept of countertransference to describe the reactions chemically dependent patients evoke in their therapists, it is clear that such intensive affective and cognitive reactions are often cogent examples of countertransference.

Levin (1991) indicates that alcoholic patients are "notorious" for the strength of the countertransference feelings they induce in therapists. He believes that countertransference is always present and refers to the negative countertransference feelings of anger, frustration, depression, and anxiety. The therapist's lack of awareness of these personal feelings can be disabling.

Countertransference (Weiss, 1994) is also associated with the tendency of medical and psychiatric departments to "inadvertently disown" the alcoholic patient, the resistance toward treating substance abusers, and the professional misconception that alcoholics and substance abusers are impossible to treat. Weiss (1994) correctly associates countertransference dynamics with the "second-class" status of alcoholic patients in relation to "bona fide" medical and psychiatric patients, and she notes that this lack of social status is often transferred to substance abuse treatment providers. Thus, institutions are vulnerable to unconscious countertransference reactions toward addicts and substance abuse in general. Weiss (1994) states that "countertransference toward the alcoholic patient can reverberate throughout an institution" (p. 409). This author indicates that alcoholics often arouse feelings of discouragement, anger, chaos, anxiety, and regression in the clinician.

Shaffer (1994) has related treatment failure to provider countertransference. He also believes that the struggle with ambivalence and addiction stimulates countertransferential hate and rage in clinicians who treat addicts. According to Shaffer (1994), "blaming patients for failing to thrive in treatment is a sophisticated form of displaying clinical hate, one expression of countertransference hate" (p. 429). Discharging patients from treatment is "typically a countertransferential act that protects clinicians from both their impulses to behave maliciously and the anxiety generated by their inability to control patient behavior patterns" (p. 431).

Recently, the author (Forrest, 1998a, 1999, 2000) examined the recondite aspects of countertransference in the psychotherapy of chemically dependent clients and prison populations. Many therapists wisely avoid working with chemically dependent persons due to a keen awareness of their personal negative feelings about and reactions to these individuals. Indeed, it is clinically and ethically important for therapists to be aware of countertransference dynamics that (1) impede the therapist's ability to function in an optimally therapeutic fashion; (2) contribute to the therapist's inability to initiate or sustain a productive psychotherapy relationship with a particular patient or subgroup; or (3) impact the process of therapy in a parataxic fashion. Therapists need to be firm in their refusal to initiate treatment relationships with persons who fall into the second category. Personal therapy and active supervision make it possible for the psychotherapist to work effectively with some patients who provoke countertransference reactions that fall within the scope of categories 1 and 3.

Substance abusers and chemically dependent patients tend to elicit countertransference reactions in the psychotherapist that are associated with matters pertaining to control, rescuing, persecution, victimizing, narcissism, competency and self-worth, impotence, rage, sexuality, and intimacy (Forrest, 1991, 1992, 1998b, 1999). These patients are frequently depressed, dysfunctional, and involved in victim roles within the family system and community when they are initially seen for treatment. It is all too easy for the psychotherapist to respond to such persons in an overdetermined, zealous, rescuing-oriented fashion. Recovering chemical dependency counselors and therapists are especially prone to experiencing this type of countertransference reaction. Overdetermined rescuing transactions on the part of the therapist may eventually provoke a role reversal situation, whereby the therapist actually becomes angry or enraged at the patient and assumes a persecutory therapeutic stance. These countertransference reactions are extremely psychonoxious and can result in relapse and suicidal acting out by the patient (Forrest, 1979). When the therapist's rescuing efforts fail, it is possible to feel frustrated and angry at the patient and then unconsciously move against the patient in a victimizing and persecuting manner. The therapist neurotically attempts to control the patient in these situations.

Many substance abusers and chemically dependent patients have an uncanny ability to feed the psychotherapist's inadequately met narcissistic needs early in the therapeutic process. During the "honeymoon" phase of therapy, the patient becomes drug abstinent, may be a model patient, and continually extols the many virtues of the psychotherapist. In sum, the patient reinforces the therapist for his or her rescuing activities. The emotional demands of the middle stages of therapy and/or relapses while in treatment often result in a rupture of the therapeutic alliance. The omnipotent status of the psychotherapist is reduced to meaninglessness by the patient. In these situations, it is absolutely imperative that the therapist avoids countertransference reactions that involve directing feelings of anger, rage, and retaliation against the patient.

The therapist is not able to control his or her chemically dependent patients, and it is the patients who must assume the lion's share of responsibility for remaining drug abstinent and maintaining a recovery program. It may be necessary for the therapist to exert control over a patient vis-à-vis hospitalization or intervention, but it is impossible, and countertransference oriented, for the clinician to attempt to control the patient. Furthermore, these patients are extremely rebellious and act out against the controlling tactics of all people whom they perceive as authority figures. Thus, it is important for the therapist to communicate verbally and behaviorally to the patient that the patient is responsible for becoming self-regulated and self-controlled within and beyond the context of the therapeutic relationship.

The chemically dependent patient and his or her family sometimes blame the psychotherapist or treatment center for relapses or continued pathologic behaviors. These stressful situations may result in feelings of failure, guilt, and shame (Hahn, 2000) and a lowered sense of professional competency in the therapist. The extremely recalcitrant patient can exacerbate feelings of incompetence and impotence in the counselor. These countertransference responses are damaging to the therapist and the therapeutic alliance. Indeed, the chemically dependent patient is capable of challenging the psychotherapist's healthy narcissism and basic sense of self-worth (Irons and Forrest, 1998; Carruth, 2000). These persons also anger the therapist by failing to keep appointments, resisting the treatment process, not taking medications, continuing to ingest alcohol and/or other drugs while in treatment, and acting out. Rage-oriented retaliations against the patient by the therapist are an example of extremely iatrogenic countertransference. Angry, hostile thoughts and fantasies about the patient are often precursors to countertransference situations that involve the therapist acting out against the patient.

Chemically dependent patients often stir countertransference reactions in the therapist that are sexually oriented or associated with intimacy or dependency issues. Chemically dependent patients and substance abusers sometimes consciously attempt to seduce the psychotherapist. It is not uncommon for these patients to dress seductively, interact with the therapist in an overtly seductive manner, or even verbally suggest to the therapist that he or she would like to engage in sexual intercourse or some other form of sexual activity with the therapist. Some of these individuals have led very promiscuous lifestyles (Forrest, 1994; Carruth, 2000). The interpersonal modus operandi of many substance abusers is pathologically sexualized.

The sexually oriented countertransference dynamics that evolve in the process of psychotherapy with chemically dependent and substance-abusing persons vary from client to client and are generally multifaceted. Most of these persons manifest sexual problems, and many fear or avoid sexual intimacy (Forrest, 1999; Wilsnack and Beckman, 1984; Wilsnack and Klassen, 1988; Stucky, 1995; Irons and Schneider, 1999). Identity disturbance is central to the psychopathology of addictive disorders. Thus, some of these patients are uncomfortable with same-sex therapists while others are conflicted in the context of an opposite-sex therapist-patient relationship. The psychotherapist needs to be sensitive to these realities and cannot permit himself or herself to become enmeshed in sexual and/or gender-oriented countertransference reactions.

Therapists sometimes become frustrated and confused about their personal feelings or reactions to the chemically dependent patient's intimacy conflicts within the explicit context of the therapeutic alliance. These individuals are very ambivalent about all close or intense human relationships. Consciously, the patient wants and needs to feel loved, close, and dependent in his or her relationship with the therapist and significant others. At preconscious and unconscious levels of awareness, the chemically dependent patient is extremely anxious and terrified by human contact and interpersonal intimacy. Early life narcissistic need and entitlement deprivation experiences have prototaxically conditioned the patient to expect to be profoundly hurt within the context of all intimate human encounters (Forrest, 1985, 1997b, 1999). Thus, the patient vacillates in his or her interpersonal movements toward, against, and away from the therapist and the therapeutic relationship. Chemically dependent patients fear a loss of self of psychosis within the context of all intimate human relationships. Identity defusion and self-system fragmentation are long-term experiential realities with which these individuals struggle (Forrest, 1997b, 1999), and which they reexperience whenever they become involved in an intimate encounter.

These patients can also be extremely demanding, dependent, and parasitic in their relationships with therapists. The psychotherapist may experience countertransference reactions in treatment relationships with such persons that involve feelings of engulfment, being trapped, and being "sucked dry." It is essential that the therapist not allow the extremely passive-dependent patient to establish a parasitic/dependency-oriented therapeutic relationship through which the psychotherapist becomes a fixated mother-object. A neurotic or false sense of intense intimacy tends to develop in psychotherapeutic relationships involving passive-dependent addicts and therapists who either are extremely dependent or allow themselves to become fixated mother-objects to the patients. The therapist can minimize this form of countertransference reaction by consistently helping the patient to be responsible for himself or herself, maintaining appropriate therapeutic boundaries, or sustaining and reinforcing limit-setting behaviors.

The severely passive-dependent substance abuser may wish to be seen in treatment several times a week, call the therapist on the telephone in the evenings or whenever he or she experiences some minimal level of dissonance, and develop an inability to make any decision without first consulting the therapist. The psychotherapist's needs for privacy and autonomy can facilitate the outcropping of various countertransference dynamics.

Therapists also experience countertransference conflicts that are associated with patients' inability to develop a basic sense of closeness, intimacy, and relatedness to the therapists. It is relatively easy for neophyte therapists to

1. blame themselves for lack of in-depth relatedness and intimacy in the psychotherapeutic relationship;
2. fail to appreciate the impact of the patients' intimacy disturbance on themselves and the development of the therapeutic alliance; and
3. respond to the patients' intimacy disturbance in a fashion that is essentially unhealthy and countertransference determined.

Therapists need to be able to accept that they cannot magically resolve or undo the chemically dependent patient's intimacy disturbance in a few therapy sessions. The patient's intimacy conflicts evolve and become real within the context of the therapeutic relationship, and this particular nexus of pathology is subject to resolution only via the process of an extended and productive therapeutic experience.

Chemically dependent or substance-abusing antisocial patients are sometimes quick to blame their therapists when they relapse or persist in pathologic patterns of behavior (Forrest, 1996). It is a simple but real fact that these individuals are difficult to treat, and some seem to be constitutionally incapable of changing or recovering. The parents and/or spouses of the patients may also blame the therapists for relapses or therapeutic failure. Attorneys, and even the legal system, can become a source of dissonance for the clinician who works with these patients (Forrest and Gordon, 1990). All of these realities impact the psychotherapist. Indeed, countertransference reactions that involve therapist self-doubting; therapist feelings of failure, inadequacy, and impotence; and basic questions about professional incompetence do occur in clinical work with chemically dependent and substance-abusing persons. Some of these patients are consciously determined to defeat the psychotherapist (Stekel, 1929; Forrest, 1999). The unconscious catagogic strivings of the patient may encompass a symbolic castration of the therapist.

Multiple relapses by the same patient or simultaneous massive regressions on the part of several patients at the same time can facilitate therapist feelings of self-doubt (Gorski and Miller, 1986; Gorski, 1991, 1992; Carruth, 2000). In these situations, the therapist may become depressive and act out a variety of countertransference reactions. Therapist reactions and transactions that are in any way governed by the talion principle are clearly destructive and therapeutically malignant. *Lex talionis* represents the most regressive and pathologic form of countertransference reaction that is associated with patient relapse/massive regression within the context of the intensive psychotherapy relationship (Forrest, 1999). The basic self-worth of the psychotherapist, as well as that of the patient, is severely damaged when this form of countertransference reaction becomes fully manifest.

COUNTERTRANSFERENCE AND COUNTERTRANSFERENCE DISTORTION

It is this author's opinion that countertransference is a natural and normal component of all psychotherapy relationships, particularly all such relationships (Glasser, 2000) with chemically dependent persons. Countertransference can be an adaptive mechanism or vehicle whereby the therapist is able to empathize with and intuitively understand the chemically dependent patient. The psychotherapist's identification process is facilitated by empathy and countertransference. Countertransference can involve all the feelings that the therapist has for the patient, and therapeutic empathy is an essential ingredient in all constructive and productive therapeutic relationships.

Empathy and countertransference are entwined. Elsewhere (Forrest, 1992) accurate empathy is defined as "the ability of a therapist to be both affectively and cognitively attuned to what the patient is currently feeling and experiencing and to communicate to the patient an understanding of these feelings" (p. 10). Empathy also reflects the ability of one person to identify with another person. In the therapeutic context, the therapist's empathy consists of his or her ability to *project* personal feelings, behaviors, cognitions, and experiential reality in order to better understand the patient.

The psychotherapeutic relationship becomes less than human and loses its efficacy when the therapist is unable to empathically relate to the patient. Countertransference contributes to the feelings, cognitions, and behaviors of the therapist that facilitate the capacity for healthy therapeutic empathy and identification. Countertransference forms the experiential being of the psychotherapist that empathically attaches to the experiential being of the patient in a fashion that becomes a vehicle for potential constructive personal growth and change upon the part of the patient, and even the therapist.

Normal and healthy countertransference can become distorted and clearly pathologic in its effect upon the patient, therapeutic relationship, and therapist. In contrast to the effects of normal and healthy countertransference, countertransference distortion impedes the development and evolution of empathy, identification, and understanding in the therapeutic relationship. The effects of countertransference distortion can be devastating to the patient and the therapeutic alliance. Overdetermined or distorted countertransference reactions involve a plethora of unhealthy and maladaptive therapist behaviors. Therapist insensitivity, scotomization, irrational thinking, anger, projection, depression, and affective conflicts constitute but a few of the destructive dynamic realities of countertransference distortion.

The major sources of countertransference-oriented conflict in chemical dependency counseling will be discussed in the following chapter. Countertransference and countertransference distortion occur on a continuum. The absence of countertransference is suggestive of a superficial, nonmeaningful, therapeutic relationship that is lacking in sufficient depth to facilitate adaptive patient change. Healthy and constructive countertransference enables the therapist to facilitate patient growth and change vis-à-vis empathy, identification, and understanding. Countertransference distortion malignantly affects the patient and the therapeutic alliance as well as the psychotherapist.

SUMMARY

The chemical dependency counseling and treatment literature includes very few references to countertransference. Historically, many chemical dependency counselors have been unfamiliar with the concept of countertransference.

Countertransference has generally not been used to explain and understand the intense emotional responses chemically dependent or substance-abusing clients often provoke in their counselors and therapists. However, virtually all experienced and professionally trained chemical dependency counselors are very familiar with the clinical experience of struggling with intense and even personally disturbing or disruptive feelings, thoughts, and impulses associated with clients and treatment relationships. These therapist reactions and responses are manifestations of countertransference.

As discussed in this chapter, the author (1979, 1992, 1994, 1997b, 1999) has examined the concept of countertransference in chemical dependency counseling at some length. Countertransference is defined in the context of intensive alcoholism psychotherapy as "the therapist's inappropriate and neurotic reactions to the patient and the psychotherapy relationship" (Forrest, 1997b, p. 84). Various other facets of countertransference in chemical dependency counseling and treatment were discussed in this chapter.

Countertransference is a natural and normal component of all psychotherapy relationships. Healthy countertransference contributes to feelings, cognitions, behaviors, and communications of the therapist that enhance the therapist's capacities for empathy, identification, and understanding. To the contrary, countertransference distortion refers to the unhealthy and overdetermined reactions of the therapist that impede the development of his or her empathy, identification, and understanding within the therapeutic encounter. Countertransference distortion harms the patient and is very often a significant factor in cases involving treatment failure.

The major problems and sources of countertransference distortion in chemical dependency counseling and psychotherapy are explored in the following chapter.

Chapter 4

Countertransference Distortion

INTRODUCTION

Countertransference contributes to the development of myriad problems and conflicts in counseling and psychotherapy relationships. Perhaps this reality influenced the early psychoanalytic efforts to eliminate all countertransference from the analyst and the psychoanalytic relationship. As noted in Chapter 1, the early Freudians were aware of the distorted or neurotic nature of countertransference in psychoanalysis and psychotherapy relationships.

Chemical dependency counseling is consistently difficult and stressful work for most counselors and clients. Counseling and psychotherapy relationships with chemically dependent or substance-abusing clients can also provide very rewarding and gratifying experiences for the counselor as well as the client. However, chemically dependent clients are generally more difficult to treat than many other patient populations (Bratter and Forrest, 1985; Levin, 1991; Weiss, 1994; Carruth, 2000), and these clients tend to evoke particular countertransference distortions in the psychotherapist. Many professional counselors and psychotherapists choose not to work with alcoholics and chemically dependent persons (Bratter, 1985; Forrest, 1999; Shaffer, 1994; Culbreth and Borders, 1999). Countertransference-oriented issues may contribute significantly to the counselor's decision to avoid treatment relationships with chemically dependent clients. Countertransference distortion may also be a significant variable in the therapist's decision to work with these clients, and countertransference directly and indirectly affects the process and outcome of all therapeutic relationships with chemically dependent persons.

In the clinical experience of the author, chemically dependent clients evoke a number of relatively predictable and consistent countertransference problems in both neophyte and experienced counselors. Each of these sources of countertransference distortion is examined in this chapter.

BASIC COUNSELOR-CLIENT "FIT"

A lack of basic counselor-client "fit" can be a primary source of countertransference distortion. Effective chemical dependency counselors are psychologically comfortable with their clients. They generally like their clients and are able to form working and productive therapeutic relationships with them. Likewise, the clients of effective chemical dependency counselors experience a basic sense of trust, respect, and emotional security in their counseling relationships. They also tend to like their counselors. These are some of the ingredients in a good counselor-client fit.

Although difficult to define and describe precisely basic counselor-client fit, it is essential that the counselor-client relationship be based upon *mutual* trust, relationship security, respect, authenticity and openness, and communication. Good counselor-client fit also contributes to the development of a working and productive therapeutic alliance as well as a mutual commitment to the recovery process. Most clinicians agree that matching clients and therapists constitutes one method of improving treatment outcomes (Pattison, 1987; Emrick, 1979, 1991; Shaffer, 1994; Carruth, 2000). A good therapeutic fit is also based upon the client's ability to communicate effectively with the counselor and to experience a basic sense of trust, respect, understanding, and lack of fear and anxiety in the counseling relationship.

Countertransference distortion develops when therapists (1) basically dislike their clients and (2) consistently feel psychologically threatened, vulnerable, and/or uncomfortable within the context of their counseling relationships with chemically dependent persons. Many therapists and counselors feel anxious and threatened by addicted clients and may consciously or unconsciously fear and disdain them. Clients soon become preconsciously and consciously aware of these internal counselor dynamics, and as a result of this awareness, the therapeutic relationship becomes progressively conflicted and dysfunctional. Needless to say, at some juncture, the therapeutic process may be terminated or ruptured as a result of countertransference distortion that evolves from a flawed counselor-client fit.

A lucid example of poor counselor-client fit involved a graduate psychology intern whom the author supervised a few years ago. After a month of attending staffings, weekly supervision and training sessions, and self-help meetings (Alcoholics Anonymous, Narcotics Anonymous), and participating in group therapy and didactic education classes, the intern began to see a few chemically dependent clients in individual psychotherapy. Following the completion of fewer than ten individual therapy sessions with these clients, this intern told the author, "I'm finding out that I really don't like alcoholics. . . .These bastards remind me of my father when he was drinking." Through the supervision process, the intern eventually decided to terminate his clinical work with chemically dependent clients.

A flawed counselor-client fit can contribute to the outcropping of various countertransference problems, including the following:

1. Counselor inability to establish meaningful and in-depth relationships with chemically dependent clients
2. Counselor failure to initiate healthy "rescuing" transactions when clinically indicated and in a timely manner
3. Therapist detachment and aloofness in sessions
4. Reciprocal anxiety and distrust
5. Counselor utilization of pathologic confrontations and persecutor roles and transactions
6. Counselor disrespect and resentment of the client
7. Counselor anger, projection, blaming, and irrational emotional responses
8. Therapist-initiated cancellations, inappropriately brief sessions, premature treatment terminations, and frequent referrals to other therapists and treatment programs

RECOGNIZING CHEMICAL DEPENDENCY

It is essential that the chemical dependency counselor be able to recognize and accurately assess chemical dependency and substance abuse. Yet, many counselors, psychologists, psychiatrists, social workers, and family therapists fail to recognize and diagnose their clients' substance use disorders (Forrest, 1978, 1998a, 2001; Weiss, 1994; Knauert, 2000). Indeed, many clinicians fail to recognize a duck when they see a duck (Forrest, 1992)! This diagnostic dilemma sometimes even pertains to experienced and skilled chemical dependency counselors.

The therapist also needs to recognize when chemical dependency or substance abuse does not exist or is of secondary relevance to the effective care of a client. Many chemically dependent clients manifest a dual diagnosis or multiple coexisting diagnoses. In this regard, recovering counselors tend to overdiagnose chemical dependency in their clients while nonrecovering clinicians tend to underdiagnose substance abuse or chemical dependency in their clients (Forrest, 1978; Lawson and Lawson, 1992; Shaffer, 1994; Culbreth and Borders, 1999).

Several years ago, it was very common for therapists to misdiagnose or fail to recognize their clients' chemical dependency. Tragically, countless numbers of persons have died from alcoholism and chemical dependency while actively engaged in therapy and being treated for depression or some other psychiatric illness.

A diversity of countertransference problems and distortions develop when the counselor fails to recognize and differentially diagnose chemical dependency or substance abuse in his or her clients (Knauert, 1979, 2000; Forrest, 1997b, 1999). An inability upon the part of the counselor to recognize consistently client chemical dependency problems early in the treatment relationship is sometimes associated with countertransference distortion related to the counselor's personal substance abuse or chemical dependency. This pattern of countertransference distortion may also be associated with present or historic chemical dependency problems in the therapist's family of origin. Whereas inadequate training, poor assessment and diagnostic skills, and a lack of clinical supervision may all contribute to a counselor's infrequent failure to recognize chemical dependency in clients, a consistent pattern of counselor misdiagnosis (underdiagnosis and/or overdiagnosis) is very often indicative of countertransference distortion.

Projection in the recovering chemical dependency counselor is also a common source of countertransference distortion in the treatment relationship (Culbreth and Borders, 1999). In these situations, the recovering counselor projects his or her personal history of drug dependence upon most, if not all, clients. These counselors also tend to perceive irrationally any drinking or substance abuse by the client or others as indicative of chemical dependency. Counselors manifesting this form of countertransference distortion may focus all of their therapeutic efforts in the area of chemical dependency and frequently fail to recognize and diagnose other coexisting significant psychiatric problems.

Underrecognizing and overrecognizing chemical dependency or substance abuse are common manifestations of countertransference distortion in chemical dependency counseling. Therapists become confused, angry, frustrated, and threatened when their clients continue to drink, relapse, or fail to improve in therapy (Carruth, 2000). Clients also manifest various unhealthy responses as a result of these therapist countertransference distortions. These countertransference problems are virtually unavoidable if the counselor fails to accurately diagnose, differentially diagnose, and recognize substance use disorders early in the treatment relationship. The following countertransference distortions are associated with accurately assessing chemical dependency:

1. Consistent pattern of underdiagnosis or overdiagnosis of chemical dependency based upon counselor denial or projection mechanisms
2. Continued substance abuse/dependency or frequent relapses by the client (or counselor)
3. Protracted "honeymoon" stage of therapy between counselor and client
4. Minimal client change related to even long-term therapy
5. Abrupt and early unilateral client treatment terminations
6. Counselor frustration, confusion, and anger after several months of unsuccessful treatment

The author frequently receives referrals from highly respected and well-trained colleagues in his community. Some of these referrals involve essentially the same dynamics:

1. The purpose of the referral is for a "substance abuse evaluation."
2. The client has been seen in individual psychotherapy two or three times per week for two or more years.
3. There has been no progress ("therapeutic stalemate") for three to six months.
4. The referring therapist now "suspects" the patient has a "drinking problem."

In each of these cases (seven cases in four years), the client had been consuming at least a pint of hard liquor per night since entering therapy! One client was actually killed in an automobile accident some four months after being evaluated by the author. He was acutely intoxicated at the time of the fatal accident. This brief case vignette provides a tragic example of countertransference distortion and the importance of accurately diagnosing chemical dependency.

RELAPSE

The process of relapse in chemical dependency counseling can both be facilitated by countertransference distortion and trigger rather extreme countertransference reactions in the counselor (Gorski and Miller, 1986; Gorski, 1991, 1992; Forrest, 1999). Counselors who *fail* to (1) recognize their clients' chemical dependency or substance abuse, (2) initiate appropriate therapeutic interventions aimed at resolving their clients' substance use disorder, or (3) maintain an ongoing addiction focus throughout the course of therapy may actually reinforce their clients' continued substance abuse or chemical dependency (Forrest, 1998a, 1999). Thus, countertransference distortion vis-à-vis repeated relapses may contribute to the demise of the therapeutic alliance or even contribute to the eventual death of the client.

Counselor verbalizations and messages that encourage or reinforce further drinking and substance abuse upon the part of the client are destructive manifestations of countertransference. Therapists who encourage their chronic alcoholic patients to attempt "controlled drinking" may be unconsciously and preconsciously killing their patients via countertransference. Counselors who routinely "give up" on their clients and are unable to intervene actively to deter or terminate a relapse may also be acting out countertransference distortion.

It is important to recognize that a relapse or multiple relapses in chemical dependency counseling can also precipitate a variety of countertransference problems. Relapse is a normal component of the process of chemical dependency counseling. However, the counselor may experience threatening feelings of professional inadequacy or incompetence, depression, anger, fear, anxiety, and guilt associated with relapse. Multiple relapses or several clients experiencing a relapse at the same time can also exacerbate countertransference. A colleague and close friend of the author recently had a client relapse and subsequently die as a result of "accidental" drug overdose. This colleague was unable to sleep or eat and was preoccupied, depressed, anxious, guilty, and unable to practice for several days after his client's death. Dr. D. experienced a possible brief countertransference psychosis following his client's relapse and subsequent death.

The following are sources of countertransference distortion associated with relapse:

1. Counselor transactions that consciously or unconsciously reinforce continued client substance abuse or dependence
2. Counselor denial of chemical dependency
3. Counselor failure to utilize treatment strategies and interventions to deter relapse or to intervene once the relapse process has been initiated
4. Counselor failure to maintain an ongoing addiction focus throughout the course of chemical dependency counseling
5. Pathologic counselor emotional reactions and control tactics
6. *Counselor relapse* or initiation of a substance use disorder

Relapses on the part of recovering chemical dependency counselors or the initiation of substance abuse by nonrecovering counselors can be manifestations of countertransference distortion. Recovering counselors are especially at risk for relapse when several of their clients simultaneously experience a relapse. Client relapse can also facilitate an emotional relapse or marked psychological disturbance in the therapist. Thus, a relapse or "massive regression" by the client may foster the outcropping of severe countertransference conflicts in the counselor (Forrest, 1997b, 1999).

It is always helpful for counselors to remember that chemically dependent clients must always assume the lion's share of responsibility for their recoveries and relapses. Relapse occurs in effective as well as ineffective therapeutic relationships with chemically dependent persons. Relapse can be a productive learning experience for both client and counselor. Countertransference distortion can affect the counselor's conscious and unconscious decisions to terminate the treatment relationship following a relapse; it may also lead the counselor to blame himself or herself and/or the client for the relapse, punish the client, or behave, think, and emote in any number of other inappropriate and psychonoxious ways (Forrest, 1992). Relapse prevention training and supervision can help the counselor resolve or better cope with these sources of countertransference distortion (Gorski, 1992; Carruth, 2000).

SEVERE COUNSELOR CHARACTER PATHOLOGY

As noted in Chapter 1, counselors and therapists are first and foremost human beings. Counselors experience a multiplicity of conflicts and problems in their personal lives. Some of these conflicts are situational and mild while others may be chronic or severe. All forms of conflict in therapists' personal lives may result in countertransference, yet severe and chronic counselor psychopathology is always a major source of countertransference distortion within the therapeutic relationship.

Countertransference problems and distortions that evolve from severe counselor character pathology rather than from the counselor's neurotic conflicts and the routine difficulties of daily living tend to be far more destructive, intense, and chronic or repetitive. Severely conflicted therapists consistently damage their clients. Indeed, countertransference distortions that stem from the counselor's severe character pathology form the basis of the process of psychonoxious psychotherapy (Truax and Carkhuff, 1967). The characterologically disturbed counselor may be chronically angry and enraged, explosive, narcissistic, manipulative and exploitive, severely depressed, sexually disturbed, and/or cognitively impaired. Many of these counselors manifest borderline personality disorder (Kernberg, 1975), antisocial personality disorder (Forrest, 1996), severe passive-aggressive personality disorder, or a severe mixed personality disorder. Recovering chemical dependency counselors may also manifest neurologic or cognitive impairments (Sena, 1993) that adversely affect their counseling relationships.

In the experience of the author, it is very difficult, if not impossible, to remediate, extinguish, or radically modify severe counselor character pathology. The chronically and severely conflicted counselor should be actively encouraged to seek employment in a more appropriate career field (Aspy et al., 2000).

Countertransference distortions that are related to severe counselor character pathology are as follows:

1. Counselor inability to establish and maintain therapeutic relationships
2. Client deterioration in therapy (persistent relapsing, suicidal acting out, or development of major affective illness)
3. Frequent suicide attempts and multiple incidents of successful suicide in clients
4. Overt hostility, blaming, and scapegoating/victimizing upon the part of the counselor

Clients of severely conflicted counselors often belittle and attack their counselors. These counseling relationships contain very little *mutual* respect, trust, empathy, and succor. It is very difficult for a client to perceive a disturbed counselor as a positive role model. Healthy identification, introjection, incorporation, and emulation do not occur in such a treatment relationship. Several years ago, the author supervised a licensed clinical social worker who was employed as a chemical dependency counselor at a comprehensive military alcohol and drug rehabilitation center. Eventually, the author learned that this counselor employed several prostitutes, operated two massage parlors, frequently engaged in sex with the wives of clients, and only worked some fifteen hours per week! Mr. M. had also experienced a brain aneurysm about fifteen years earlier and prior to completing his graduate degree in social work. He was disliked and disrespected by his clients as well as other staff members. Following a plethora of legal procedures, Mr. M. was terminated from his position, and the Federal Civil Service System effectively ended his career as a chemical dependency counselor.

BOUNDARY VIOLATIONS
AND SEXUAL ACTING OUT

Boundary violations and sexual exploitation of clients are facilitated vis-à-vis countertransference distortion, which is almost always very closely related to counselor character pathology (Irons and Schneider, 1999). Most studies indicate that less than 10 percent of psychiatrists, clinical psychologists, and social workers engage in sexual activities with their patients (Pope, 1986; Dove, 1995). It is reasonable to expect that a similar percentage of chemical dependency counselors also become sexually involved with their clients. Boundary violations or sexual liaisons between a counselor and client are psychologically damaging to the client, unethical, and clinically inappropriate.

Boundary violations and sexual abuse of clients are forms of countertransference distortion that evolve from the counselor's unresolved identity and sexual pathology, impulse control deficits, low self-esteem, and underlying feelings of inadequacy. Boundary violations involve any inappropriate touching, fondling, or sexual transactions between the counselor and client. The counselor is ultimately responsible for setting and maintaining appropriate boundaries in the therapeutic relationship. Although a small percentage of clients may attempt to initiate sexual activities or other boundary violations with the counselor, the counselor is always responsible for the professional management, containment, termination, and resolution of these transactions (Forrest, 1998a).

Most counselors and therapists are knowledgeable about the ethical parameters of their relationships with clients, a few are not, and others are characterologically unable to manage the ethical demands and requirements of professional counseling and psychotherapy. Several months ago the author was asked to provide expert witness testimony in a court case that involved a licensed CAC (certified addictions counselor) professional chemical dependency counselor who sexually assaulted a client. The counselor actually had sexual intercourse with his client while she was in a hospital being detoxified from alcohol! When questioned about the unethical aspects of this behavior during a deposition, the counselor reported that he *now* realized that it was "unethical" for him to engage in sexual intercourse with his client because "I'm a married man." Tragically, the counselor in this case had neither the training and education in ethics nor the personal integrity to avoid boundary and sexual violations with clients.

Indicators of countertransference distortion that are related to boundary violations and sexual acting out include the following:

1. Compulsive touching, hugging, or other forms of physical contact between the counselor and client (usually counselor initiated)
2. Counselor preoccupation with the client (e.g., verbalizations, dreams, obsessive ideation, etc.)
3. Extended counseling sessions and/or scheduling clients for frequent crisis or additional therapy sessions
4. Failure to bill clients for sessions
5. Conscious sexual feelings, ideation, and fantasies before, during, and after counseling sessions
6. Inappropriate *verbal* boundary violations and sexual acting out by the counselor
7. Inability to discuss openly and share sexual reactions to clients with the clinical supervisor or in appropriate clinical settings (staff training and supervision sessions, etc.)
8. Acute and/or chronic marital discord or severe relationship disturbance with significant others
9. Generalized insensitivity and lack of awareness pertaining to feelings, needs, and boundaries of others
10. Prior history of sexual acting out and impulse control problems

Finally, it is also important to point out that boundary violations and sexual acting out can occur on a verbal level between the therapist and client (Irons and Schneider, 1999). Although this behavior may be generally less abusive and destructive to the client, it is nonetheless a salient component of severe countertransference distortion. Countertransference distortions may be reflected in the counselor's verbal style, through jokes and cursing, and by a global pattern of verbal interactions with a client. Verbal boundary violations and verbal sexual acting out are countertransference problems that adversely affect the client and the therapeutic relationship.

Sexual acting out between clients and persons other than the counselor can also result in countertransference or be facilitated by countertransference distortion. Clients in therapy groups sometimes develop sexual relationships with one another. These liaisons can provoke or result from intense countertransference distortion. Counselor control tactics or avoidance and denial of these forms of client sexual acting out are often indicative of countertransference distortion.

TERMINATION, SUICIDE, AND RUPTURE OF THE THERAPEUTIC ALLIANCE

The termination phase of chemical dependency counseling (Forrest, 1997b, 1998a) is rarely addressed in the substance abuse treatment and rehabilitation literature. Suicide and rupture of the therapeutic alliance are also topics that are not elucidated in the chemical dependency treatment literature. However, therapy termination, successful suicide and/or attempted suicide, and rupture of the therapeutic alliance are all transactions that can serve as catalysts for countertransference in the chemical dependency counselor. These transactions consistently trigger countertransference reactions in the chemical dependency counselor, and they may also be indirectly facilitated by the countertransference distortions of the counselor. The death or physical illness of a client also may stir intense countertransference in the therapist.

Terminating the therapeutic relationship can stir feelings of loss, abandonment, separation anxiety, and grief in the counselor as well as the client. As noted earlier (Forrest, 1999), therapists also experience conflicted and sometimes neurotic (countertransference distortion) feelings about "letting go" of their patients. Efficacious and successful counseling relationships can be just as difficult for the counselor and client to terminate as conflicted and unproductive therapeutic relationships.

The following sources of countertransference distortion are frequently related to the process of terminating the counseling relationship:

1. Avoiding or failing to develop treatment termination strategies (plan)
2. Fostering client dependency on the counselor or counselor codependency
3. Counselor depression
4. Counselor failure to maintain an addiction focus, which can result in unconscious sabotage of the client's treatment success vis-à-vis relapse
5. Counselor failure to explore openly and consistently self-oriented as well as client-oriented feelings and reactions to the process of termination counseling

As touched upon earlier in this chapter, countertransference is always precipitated by suicidal acting out or a successful suicide by a client. The therapist can be expected to feel anxious, threatened, depressed, sad, grieved, helpless, and vulnerable when his or her clients act out suicidally. These countertransference distortions evoke suicidal acting out by clients:

1. Counselor failure to assess accurately client depression and/or suicide risk potential (plan or intent)
2. Counselor failure to implement adequate suicide prevention strategies
3. Unconscious, preconscious, or even overt counselor reinforcement of client suicidal intent and ideation
4. Counselor relapse, decompensation, or other extreme emotional reactions to client suicidal acting out

An acute rupture of the therapeutic alliance may also be partially caused by countertransference distortion or result in an acute countertransference reaction. Abrupt, premature, and unilateral (client-initiated) ruptures in therapeutic relationships almost always involve countertransference dynamics. These terminations can be especially upsetting to both the counselor and client. Chemically dependent clients are especially prone to a pattern of abruptly and unilaterally terminating treatment. Therapeutic alliances with these persons (Levin, 1991) are almost always relatively fragile, difficult, and precarious. However, some chemical dependency counselors are also more prone than other therapists to acting out countertransference distortions that cause abrupt, premature, inappropriate, and unilateral ruptures in their therapeutic relationships.

A persistent pattern of acute and conflicted ruptures in the therapeutic alliance can be related to the following countertransference problems: (1) inadequate counselor skills and lack of treatment progress, (2) poor counselor-client "fit," and (3) affective disturbance (usually depression) or impulse control problems in the counselor. However, it must be noted that in chemical dependency counseling, most ruptures in the therapeutic alliance are the product of client relapse. The therapist's countertransference reactions to client relapse may also be intense and involve pathologic anger, depression, feelings of inadequacy and professional incompetence, anxiety and stress, sleep disturbance and physiologic symptoms, relapse and/or the initiation of substance abuse, or even confused thinking and acting out. Counselors often attempt to initiate more control over their chemically dependent clients when clients experience a relapse.

The "normal" process of terminating therapy, suicide or suicidal acting out, and a rupture of the therapeutic alliance are all concrete and lucid examples of finality. Human beings generally experience conflict and intense emotions when significant relationships end. This is true regardless of the specific circumstances surrounding a meaningful relationship termination. Although a successful suicide or suicide attempt by a client will provoke a quantitatively and qualitatively different countertransference reaction in the therapist than a successful, bilateral psychotherapy termination, both forms of relationship termination can be expected to provoke countertransference.

The counseling, psychotherapy (Glasser, 1965; 2000), and the chemical dependency treatment literature has failed to explore adequately countertransference-oriented distortions associated with the various processes of therapy termination, suicide or suicidal acting out, and rupture of the therapeutic alliance. The death, physical illness, or geographical relocation of a client may result in countertransference. Countertransference and parataxic distortion can also facilitate and/or result from these processes.

FEES, BILLING, SCHEDULING, AND OTHER PRACTICAL ISSUES

Countertransference problems often develop as a result of the practical dimensions of the counselor-client relationship (Slakter, 1987; Tansey and Burke, 1989). Matters pertaining to money and counselor fee management are especially apt to provoke countertransference problems. Client failure to pay for sessions, late payments, problems associated with insurance billing and reimbursements, and problems with managed care providers tend to generate countertransference. The counselor's sense of basic security is often closely associated with his or her ability to earn a living, and, thus, client transactions and behaviors that threaten the basic security operations of the counselor generate strong countertransference reactions.

Arranging client appointments and scheduling sessions can also provoke countertransference problems. Most counselors are flexible and willing to schedule therapy sessions at times that are convenient for the client as well as the counselor. Likewise, most clients show up for scheduled sessions and call to reschedule or notify the counselor if they are unable to keep a scheduled appointment. Clients are also usually on time for their counseling sessions. However, a significant number of clients do not show up for sessions and/or repeatedly cancel sessions or arrive late for their appointments. Chemically dependent clients also come to their therapy sessions intoxicated, relapse, and unilaterally drop out of or terminate therapy. All of these situations inconvenience the counselor and may also prove costly for both the counselor and the client. These situations can inconvenience other clients and staff and have a disruptive influence on the counselor's entire practice. Countertransference reactions to such processes often involve intensified counselor feelings of anger, resentment, frustration, and inadequacy, as well as a diminished sense of personal efficacy.

Vulnerability to countertransference distortion is also related to the therapist's relationships and interactions with office staff and colleagues. A parataxic relationship with the office secretary or a professional colleague can precipitate a multiplicity of countertransference reactions. The office secretary is usually responsible for scheduling or rescheduling client therapy sessions, answering phone calls, billing, filing insurance forms, collecting fees, and developing a supportive and caring emotional rapport with the office staff. Office managers and accountants are responsible for billing policies, collection of fees, management of insurance matters, tax preparation and payment, and counselor reimbursement. Professional colleagues interact with the counselor on a daily basis, are periodically "on call" for the counselor, attend regular staff meetings, help shape and determine office procedures and policies, and may be rather intimately involved in many of the professional and social activities of the counselor. It is rather obvious and understandable that countertransference distortion may evolve from and/or cause various conflicts in any or all of these realms.

Countertransference problems related to fees, billing, and other office-related practical issues include the following:

1. Counselor preoccupation with monetary aspects of practice
2. Lack of consistent fee structure and billing policy
3. Persistent conflict associated with scheduling clients
4. Repetitive difficulties with secretaries, colleagues, and other office personnel

Counselors and therapists can eliminate most sources of countertransference distortion associated with the office milieu simply by developing and maintaining *consistent* policies pertaining to fee structure, billing, scheduling, hiring and termination of employees, vacations and holidays, insurance, sick leave, salary, staff remuneration and raises, and so forth. The selection of office staff and collegial associates is key to minimizing countertransference problems in the office. However, the practice of chemical dependency counseling, as with all mental health work, is emotionally demanding and stressful. The therapeutic milieu is simply less stressful and less likely to precipitate intense countertransference problems when the office staff is comprised of bright, socially adroit, highly trained, experienced, motivated, and relatively well-adjusted individuals.

THE PROCESS OF DAILY LIVING

Countertransference distortions and problems can be precipitated by the basic process of daily living. The counselor's global adjustment style and internal frame of reference are continuously being shaped and changed by the experiences of life.

The life of the psychotherapist includes relative ups and downs and periodic crises or even devastating personal experiences. Divorce; the death of a spouse, parent, child, or significant other; illness and health problems; job loss; aging; or financial difficulties are but a few of the realities of daily living that can significantly effect the emotional well-being and countertransference reactions of the counselor. The coping mechanisms, skills, and strength of the counselor are continuously being tested vis-à-vis the process of daily living. It is highly unrealistic to expect the counselor to remain perpetually unaffected and countertransference free in his or her responses to the process of daily living. Thus, the psychotherapist is always "more simply human than otherwise."

It may be relatively easy to overlook that seemingly pleasant, positive, or life-enhancing personal experiences on the part of the counselor also potentially affect countertransference. Although painful losses and destructive personal life experiences generally result in more malignant counselor countertransference distortions, seemingly positive and rewarding life experiences can also cause significant countertransference problems. For example, the experience of falling in love or getting married may diminish the therapist's emotional availability and attachment receptiveness to clients.

Countertransference distortions that can be associated with the process of daily living include (1) acute or situational dysfunction and disturbance in the counselor and (2) chronic distortion associated with a particular chronic living problem with which the counselor struggles. Acute or situational living problems usually result in acute and time-related countertansference problems. A chronic living problem predictably results in a relatively specific area of chronic countertransference distortion. For example, the counselor who manifests a severe and chronic medical condition such as multiple sclerosis, lupus, or AIDS will usually experience persistent countertransference distortions that may be exacerbated by select clients.

Countertransference distortion and problems can be associated with virtually every facet of the counselor-client therapeutic relationship. Indeed, countertransference and various types and degrees of countertransference distortion color and shape every counseling relationship. Effective counselors and psychotherapists are consistently able to establish and maintain therapeutic relationships that are minimally affected by countertransference distortion.

Weiss (1994) has developed the following table of common countertransference reactions in psychotherapy with alcoholics (see Table 4.1). Readers may find the information included in this table to be quite helpful in their efforts to identify personal countertransference dynamics and reactions.

SUMMARY

Countertransference and/or countertransference distortion are central ingredients in the process of career choice and career development for many counselors and psychotherapists. Many chemical dependency counselors are themselves recovering alcoholics and substance abusers. Perhaps most chemical dependency counselors have been parented by chemically dependent parents or come from families of origin that include several alcoholics and/or chemically dependent persons. The spouses or children of these counselors also sometimes have substance abuse problems. All of these realities are fertile sources of counselor countertransference distortion.

TABLE 4.1. Common Countertransference Reactions in Alcohol-Focused Psychotherapy and Related Patient Dynamics

Clinician Responses	Patient Behavior/Examples	Alcohol Symptoms	Psychodynamics
Stood up Hurt Rejected Bewildered Fear of abandonment	Erratic attendance	Unreliability due to physical problems of intoxication, withdrawal	Inconsistency in object relations Guilt over drinking Ambivalence over giving up drinking
Conned Confused Deceived Exploited Angry	Concealing alcohol Misrepresenting use of other doctors, clinics Using treatment only to acquire financial or economic entitlements	Alibis required to maintain drinking Needs to manage anxiety and irritability Drinking interferes with ability to work	Replays traumatic patterns Needs to split treatment Relates with part objects
Policeman Angry Punitive Sadistic Guilty	Repeated disregard for standards, pushing clinician to enforce rigid policies	Continues alcohol use due to physical dependence Disregards consequences of actions	Provokes punishment due to guilt Lacks ego control/structure (cannot manage instincts)
Bored Loss of interest Feeling shut out Sleepy	Grandiosity Repetitive speech Lack of affect Soliloquies	Lack of experience in relationships while sober	Relates to therapist as self-object Grandiosity masks fragile self
Hopeless Helpless Impotent as helper Devalued	Denial of illness Continued drinking Sabotaging treatment	Physical dependence Repeated intoxication Advanced medical problems	Denial Faulty thinking: sees permanent flaws in self Depressive: lack of optimism Uses hopelessness to rationalize drinking
Overwhelmed Depleted Drained	Frequent calls Suicide attempts Requests for Rx Requests for additional services	Chronic use Physical dependency Feels overwhelmed by decreased alcohol	Ego deficits: cannot manage internal affects Dependency

47

TABLE 4.1 *(continued)*

Clinician Responses	Patient Behavior/Examples	Alcohol Symptoms	Psychodynamics
Charmed Intense warmth Desires closeness Physical attraction Loss of boundaries	Seductive behavior (glances, dress, comments) Flattering therapist Idealizing treatment	Intoxication: diminishes inhibitions/boundaries Sobriety: overwhelms patient with new states	Seeks merger to overcome aloneness Regression from differentiated state
Panic Guilty, anxious Fears own reputation will be destroyed Fears patient will be destroyed	Failure to get medical care High-risk behavior (casual sex, physical or sexual abuse)	Serious medical sequelae Lack of judgment Blackouts Impaired cognition Nutritional deficiencies	Denial and grandiosity Guilt, self-destructiveness Ego deficits in self-care
Sympathy Overconcern Overresponsible Rescuer fantasies	Emphasizing pain Conveying helplessness	Depression (organic) Patient isolation due to alcoholic behavior Problems with work, finances, and family	Rescue fantasies Dependency Wish for maternal caretaking
Positive regard Likes patient Appropriate concern Genuine interest Feels hopeful	Participation in AA Regular attendance in treatment program Conveys genuine involvement with therapist and others	Sobriety Adequate medical care and nutrition Improved thinking Recovery with work and family	Internalize group function of AA Character growth through twelve steps Internalize structure of therapy/therapist

Source: Weiss, R. H., 1994, pp. 414-415.

This chapter examined the major countertransference problems, sources of countertransference distortion, and countertransference dynamics in chemical dependency counseling. Countertransference distortions in chemical dependency counseling are frequently a result of the following:

1. Poor counselor-client "fit"
2. Poor counselor assessment, diagnostic, and differential diagnosis skills
3. The relapse process
4. Severe counselor character pathology
5. Counselor boundary violations and sexual abuse of clients
6. Termination, suicide, and rupture of the therapeutic alliance
7. Counselor management of fees, billing, scheduling, and other practical issues
8. The process of daily living

Relatively specific countertransference problems related to each of these eight areas were identified and discussed. Weiss's (1994) table of common countertransference reactions in alcohol-focused psychotherapy and related patient dynamics was also included in this chapter.

Countertransference contributes to the development of various conflicts and problems in chemical dependency counseling. However, the concept of countertransference is poorly understood in the chemical dependency treatment field, and this topic is rarely discussed in the chemical dependency treatment literature. Chemically dependent clients are especially difficult to treat within the context of counseling and psychotherapy relationships (Levin, 1991; Weiss, 1994; Forrest, 1997b; Carruth, 2000), and these clients tend to evoke particular countertransference reactions in counselors. This chapter includes one of the first in-depth discussions of the primary countertransference conflicts that chemical dependency counselors experience in their therapeutic relationships with substance-abusing and chemically dependent clients.

Although countertransference and various forms and degrees of countertransference distortion shape and affect every counseling relationship, optimally effective counselors and psychotherapists are consistently able to build therapeutic relationships that are minimally affected by countertransference distortion (Glasser, 2000). Effective therapists also manifest an uncanny ability to utilize countertransference as a constructive vehicle for developing adaptive client growth and change as well as self-growth and change.

Countertransference conflicts are very commonly associated with treatment relationships involving polydrug-dependent clients, clients manifesting concurrent severe psychiatric illness (Bellack, 2000), and those presenting with antisocial personality disorder or other severe personality disorders. Chemical dependency counselors need to develop extensive clinical experience with these various patient subpopulations to minimize countertransference distortions and conflicts (Forrest, 1996, 2000).

Chapter 5

Resolution and Management
of Countertransference

INTRODUCTION

As noted in earlier chapters, countertransference generally impedes the process of constructive and effective psychotherapy. Indeed, clinicians have historically been trained to avoid or limit the conscious and even unconscious expression of personal experiences, feelings, and cognitions within the context of the therapeutic encounter. Classical psychoanalysis and other schools of counseling and psychotherapy tend to view countertransference as a destructive influence on the therapeutic process. However, there is growing realization in all modern schools of counseling and psychotherapy that countertransference can potentially enhance the process and effectiveness of psychotherapy (Glasser, 1965, 2000).

Countertransference is a basic component in all counseling and psychotherapy relationships (Forrest, 1997b; 1999). Countertransference impacts the therapeutic process and outcome in a multiplicity of constructive as well as destructive ways. Thus, it is essential that chemical dependency counselors understand the concept of countertransference and develop a personal awareness of the dynamics of countertransference. It is very unrealistic as well as countertherapeutic for the chemical dependency counselor to attempt to eliminate countertransference from the counseling relationship. However, it is imperative that chemical dependency counselors be able to resolve and manage countertransference distortions in order to be consistently effective in their treatment efforts. Counselors need to be able to identify, resolve or neutralize, and manage all sources of countertransference-oriented conflict within the context of the therapeutic relationship.

The resolution and effective management of countertransference distortion in chemical dependency counseling is not easily accomplished. However, this is a more realistic and clinically appropriate counseling goal than the historic goal of removing all countertransference from the treatment relationship. This chapter provides several practical methods and alternatives for resolving and managing countertransference in chemical dependency counseling. Chemical dependency counselors and chemical dependency treatment programs need to incorporate these alternatives for resolving and managing sources of countertransference conflict into their basic plan of daily or regular operations. Strategies for coping with institutional and systemic countertransference are also elucidated in this chapter.

COUNSELOR SELECTION, EDUCATION, AND TRAINING

Traditional counselor training programs attempt to select bright, well-adjusted, sensitive, and "therapeutic" counselor trainees. Unfortunately, very few professional counselor training programs provide specific and comprehensive training and education in the area of chemical dependency counseling. This is also true with regard to traditional psychology, social work, marriage and family counseling, and psychiatry training programs. Comprehensive chemical dependency treatment programs also tend to provide very limited training, education, and supervision experiences for chemical dependency counselors in training.

The counselor selection process for most chemical dependency counselors has historically been random, or perhaps archaic, at best. Prior to the past few years, most chemical dependency counselors have somehow been "selected" to treat substance abusers and chemically dependent persons as a result of their personal struggles with drug addiction and following months or sometimes years of personal recovery. Most clinicians in the chemical dependency treatment field have not been "selected" for professional undergraduate or graduate counseling training or even employment in this field as a result of personal characteristics such as intelligence, integrity, character structure and personality makeup, ethics and morality, responsibility, empathy, or very general therapeutic qualities such as leadership or communication skills.

Counselor selection is a viable method for reducing and managing countertransference problems in chemical dependency counseling *before* counselors actually begin to treat clients. The identification and elimination of inappropriate and unsuitable chemical dependency counselor trainees eventually results in the elimination of a significant source of countertransference problems within the field of chemical dependency counseling and treatment.

Counselor selection is intimately and interactively related to the processes of counselor education and training. Nonetheless, chemical dependency counselors need to be *selected* for involvement in structured and intensive chemical dependency training and education programs based upon the quantitative and qualitative assessment of such personal characteristics as

1. relative absence of personal psychopathology;
2. cognitive functioning, abilities, and absence of gross brain impairment;
3. open-mindedness and capacity for training, education, and supervision;
4. prosocial cognitive and interpersonal style;
5. effective communication skills;
6. responsibility;
7. basic sense of morality and ethics;
8. social skills;
9. therapeutic qualities; and
10. ability to function effectively with chemically dependent persons.

It should also be noted that counselor trainees are not ipso facto appropriate candidates for chemical dependency counseling as a function of simply having earned an undergraduate, a graduate, or a medical degree in one of the behavioral science areas (psychology, counseling, social work, medicine, etc.).

The didactic education and experiential or clinical training of chemical dependency counselors together constitute another method for reducing countertransference problems in the chemical dependency treatment field. Education and training experiences foster counselor understanding, awareness, insight, and skill building that can help deter the manifestation of countertransference problems in actual clinical practice. Effective professional chemical dependency counselors have educational backgrounds that encompass more than simply ten to thirty years of personal substance abuse/dependence, a state certificate to provide "drug counseling" services, a college degree, or training as a health professional (Culbreth and Borders, 1999).

Chemical dependency counselors need to complete didactic educational training programs that include undergraduate- and graduate-level college course work in the areas of

1. abnormal psychology and psychopathology,
2. theories of personality,
3. models and theories of addiction,
4. theories of counseling and psychotherapy,
5. group therapy techniques,
6. professional ethics,
7. differential diagnosis and assessment,
8. research methods and statistics, and
9. basic pharmacology.

Professional chemical dependency counselors also need to complete ongoing *clinical* training programs (practicum, fieldwork placements, and internships) that involve 1,000 to 2,000 hours of actual supervised work experience in a chemical dependency treatment center and/or a psychiatric hospital. Trainees in these settings need to be actively involved in weekly staffings and training sessions as well as workshops and receive weekly individual clinical supervision.

During the decades of the 1970s and 1980s, many chemical dependency treatment programs throughout the United States "promoted" or somehow magically transformed patients into counselors after the patients had been sober/drug abstinent for a few weeks or months (Culbreth and Borders, 1999). These "neophyte" chemical dependency counselors were soon employed by the treatment agency and eventually licensed by the state as "certified alcohol and drug counselors." In general, this model of counselor selection, education, and training is grossly inadequate, inappropriate, and ethically flawed. Counselors and treatment facilities who routinely utilized this model often provided substandard patient care, were guilty of malpractice and/or ethical violations and involved in frequent lawsuits, and ultimately may have been largely responsible for the erosion of chemical dependency treatment services throughout the United States. All of these matters are intimately related to countertransference.

The process of counselor selection, education, and training is ongoing and unending. Counselor education and training is not concluded when the counselor obtains a state license or completes a graduate degree (Aspy et al., 2000). Likewise, the counselor selection process remains open and is always changing and evolving. The professional chemical dependency counselor needs to view the processes of selection, education, and training as lifelong or career-enduring methods for enhancing personal growth and professional skills as well as for resolving and managing countertransference distortion.

COUNSELOR SUPERVISION

Counselor supervision represents perhaps the single most effective method for resolving and managing countertransference. The supervision process is an extension of the processes of counselor selection, education, and training. Most professionally trained chemical dependency counselors and other health professionals (psychologists, psychiatrists, social workers, and family and marriage therapists) receive some supervision during the course of their didactic and clinical education and training experiences. Many of these clinicians have received inadequate direct supervision. The quantity and quality of their supervisory experiences may be insufficient to resolve personal sources of countertransference distortion. Furthermore, many counselors do not remain in direct clinical supervision once they have completed graduate training, a formal chemical dependency counselor training program, or following their state licensure/certification as a CAC.

Counselor trainees should be involved in weekly individual and group supervision throughout the course of their clinical training. Thus, each counselor trainee would receive a minimum of two hours of weekly individual and group supervision throughout the course of all practicum experience internships, fieldwork, and agency placements. This supervision model provides trainees with ongoing opportunities for self-exploration and self-examination, discussion, feedback, and concrete clinical teaching and learning experiences relative to all facets of countertransference.

It is imperative that educators and supervisors of counselors be experienced, well-trained, and clinically skilled in the realms of chemical dependency supervision, treatment, and assessment. The preparation of effective chemical dependency counselors includes ongoing supervision with well-trained, sensitive, knowledgeable, and experienced *supervisors.* Healthy and optimal supervisory relationships transcend "the blind leading the blind" supervisory model that has all too frequently been the reality of supervision within the context of many chemical dependency treatment programs. Again, it is essential that undergraduate and graduate counseling, psychology, psychiatry, social work, and chemical dependency education and training programs employ *supervisors and faculty members who are experienced, well-trained, and skilled in chemical dependency treatment, assessment, and supervision.*

Supervision provides the chemical dependency counselor trainee with repeated opportunities to explore personal feelings, beliefs, attitudes, and reactions to self, clients, significant others, and therapeutic relationships. Clinical supervisors help trainees examine and resolve their feelings of anger, confusion, depression, resentment, and anxiety or fear that evolve vis-à-vis the therapeutic alliance. Sexual fantasies and impulses, countertransferential hatred, feelings of inadequacy, and other countertransference reactions and dynamics can be better understood, recognized, and resolved or managed more effectively within the context of the supervisor-counselor trainee relationship. Supervisors help counselor trainees to more fully understand themselves, their clients, and the many vicissitudes of counseling relationships.

The supervisory process per se often becomes a fertile ground for the development of countertransference. Evolving awareness and exploration of the various origins and sources of supervisor-trainee countertransference within the context of the supervisory relationship constitutes another very powerful experiential method for resolving and managing trainee-client or institutionally generated sources of countertransference.

Group supervision is also an efficacious method for developing awareness and understanding of as well as for processing, resolving, and managing countertransference. The group process is especially conducive to countertransference and multiple countertransference reactions. Also, the feedback and interactive dynamics of the group process foster experiential awareness, learning, and insight related to a plethora of countertransference-oriented issues.

Counselors and psychotherapists need to be involved in some form of supervisory relationship for the duration of their clinical work. The successful completion of a doctoral degree in clinical psychology, obtaining a professional license to practice social work or substance abuse counseling, or certification as a psychiatrist or even psychoanalyst is not tantamount to the end of the need for personal supervision. Countertransference dynamics and distortion are forever components of the psychotherapeutic process. Countertransference is an ever-present, evolving component of the counseling relationship. Thus, the most skilled and effective counselors and therapists will recognize these realities and remain engaged in some form of ongoing supervision (Forrest, 1997b; Culbreth and Borders, 1999; Glasser, 2000).

The author has provided direct clinical supervision for many counselors and therapists over the past twenty-five years while continuing to receive periodically personal supervision from colleagues. Supervision is a very powerful tool for resolving and managing countertransference distortion and countertransference-oriented sources of conflict. Counselor trainees need to be involved in therapeutically facilitative supervisory relationships, and they also need to be taught that supervision is an integral and *ongoing* component of the practice of counseling and psychotherapy from the beginning until the end of a counselor's professional career.

PERSONAL THERAPY

As indicated in Chapter 1, the early psychoanalysts (Freud, 1961/1910; Fenichel, 1945) emphasized the destructive and undesirable impact of countertransference upon the psychoanalytic process. Freud (1961/1910) proposed that the psychoanalyst undergo a rather lengthy personal analysis in order to better consciously recognize and resolve countertransference material. Contemporary psychoanalytic training programs continue to require their candidates to undergo 400 to 600 hours of personal psychoanalysis in order to become certified psychoanalysts and to practice psychoanalytically oriented psychotherapy. Personal analysis is currently felt to be a viable method for developing and fostering the analyst's awareness and understanding of countertransference dynamics as well as a tool for resolving and managing countertransference problems.

Traditional counselor education and therapist training programs do not require trainees to complete 400 to 600 hours of personal analysis or therapy in order to receive their graduate degrees or certificates. Likewise, state licensing boards for psychologists, social workers, and professional counselors do not require candidates for licensure to complete a specified number of hours in personal therapy or counseling.

Counselor educators, clinical supervisors, and board licensure members generally seem to view the idea of personal therapy as a training and certification requirement or prerequisite with ambivalence. However, counselor education and other therapist training programs have always encouraged trainees to seek personal counseling "if or when they feel they need it," and increasing numbers of training programs are actually requiring students to undergo personal counseling in order to fulfill the requirements for a graduate degree. Personal counseling or therapy experiences have always been at least a secondary or tertiary component of traditional counselor education training programs vis-à-vis practicum, internships, group dynamics courses, and fieldwork experiences.

Personal therapy can be viewed as a rather logical extension of the counselor selection, education, training, and supervision processes. The counselor trainee's involvement in personal counseling or therapy is a direct extension of supervison and the supervisory relationship. Although some clinical supervision models do not envision supervision as therapy and do not advocate that supervisors attempt to develop formal counseling and psychotherapy relationships with supervisees/trainees (Hess, 1980), most clinicians would agree that all effective supervisor-trainee relationships involve many therapeutic (counselor-client) characteristics. The supervision-as-therapy training model obviously provides direct personal therapy experience for counselor trainees.

The author generally recommends that personal therapy and supervision be viewed as separate and relatively distinct clinical processes. Both are very useful in the recognition, resolution, and management of countertransference. Counselor trainees should be referred for personal therapy and/or be required to be involved in ongoing therapy when it becomes apparent to their clinical supervisors and educators that they (1) manifest significant personal psychopathology and/or (2) are experiencing *repetitive* and *clinically significant* countertransference-oriented conflicts within the context of counseling, supervisory, peer, or interpersonal relationships. When a counselor trainee is mandated to counseling, the trainee's therapist needs to be able to communicate openly and honestly with the supervisor (and possibly other counselor training faculty) relative to the trainee's progress and change in therapy. Severely disturbed counselor trainees and trainees who are unable to modify and resolve marked countertransference-oriented psychopathology need to be disengaged from the counselor training program and perhaps encouraged to seek a career outside of the counseling field.

Supervision provides an advanced or sophisticated level of training, education, and intervention that is designed to resolve and manage countertransference. Personal therapy provides a significantly more intensive, in-depth, focused, and resolution-oriented method for ameliorating countertransference distortion. Therapy is more specifically aimed at uncovering and resolving the intrapersonal and interpersonal sources of countertransference.

Recovering chemically dependent counselor trainees sometimes experience a "massive regression" (Forrest, 1978, 1999) or "relapse" (Gorski and Miller, 1986; Gorski, 1992; Carruth, 2000), returning to active alcoholism or chemical dependency, after becoming involved in a professional counselor training program. These individuals must be required to enter therapy and to begin an appropriate treatment regimen immediately, and their suitability for continued involvement in the counselor training program needs to be continually assessed and monitored by staff and supervisors. Many of these individuals simply are not appropriate candidates for the counseling and psychotherapy professions. Recovering persons need to have established and maintained at least three to five years of uninterrupted total alcohol/drug abstinence *before* they are considered for admission into a professional counselor education training program.

It may also become apparent to supervisors and faculty that some nonrecovering counselor trainees manifest chemical dependency and/or a significant substance use disorder. These individuals must also be required to enter therapy or a treatment program, establish alcohol/drug abstinence, and resolve their major conflicts in order to continue in a professional chemical dependency counselor training program. These trainees also need to be monitored closely by supervisors and faculty. They should be encouraged to continue in an ongoing recovery regimen following the completion of formal counselor training and certification.

Counselor trainees should be encouraged to enter psychotherapy at any point in their lives when they are significantly conflicted. Trainees also need to be encouraged to consider entering personal therapy whenever they are unable to resolve or effectively manage countertransference reactions within the context of their supervisory relationships. Therapy is a lifelong or career-enduring option for the counselor in his or her efforts to resolve and manage countertransference.

INSTITUTIONAL AND SYSTEMIC COUNTERTRANSFERENCE

Countertransference reactions to chemical dependency occur in institutions and health care systems as well as in the context of counselor-client relationships. Hospital emergency room staff notoriously disdain working with alcoholics and drug addicts. Physicians, psychiatrists, psychologists, social workers, and nurses have generally avoided treating chemically dependent persons. Institutions tend to manifest countertransference reactions toward chemical dependency that involve denial, disowning, and devaluation (Weiss, 1994).

The chemically dependent person is a second-class patient. Chemical dependency treatment personnel tend to be perceived as second-class health care providers. The institutional space allotted for these treatment services is often limited or relegated to an off-site location. Insurance companies and managed care organizations seem to make every effort to limit or deny reimbursement for chemical dependency treatment services. Hospital and mental health administrators are less than enthusiastic about including chemical dependency treatment units in their facilities, and health service providers generally believe that alcoholics and substance abusers are "impossible" to treat.

Institutional and systemic countertransference are significant forces in all systems and institutions: schools, hospitals, the military, churches, the government, and the penal system. Countertransference reactions in institutions and systems often take the form of authoritarianism, racism, and prejudice. Yet, these reactions are to be expected and not perceived as unique to the chemical dependency treatment field. Countertransference permeates every facet of human interaction and influences institutional and systemic behavior as well as dyadic forms of human relatedness.

One major challenge facing professional chemical dependency counselors and drug education specialists is that of resolving or more effectively managing institutional and systemic countertransference distortion. How can this complex and difficult challenge be met by counselors and educators? Although there are no quick, simple, or easy solutions to the multifaceted problems of institutional and systemic countertransference in the chemical dependency treatment field, beginning points, resolution and change-oriented alternatives, and pathways to change do exist. Individual chemical dependency counselors and drug educators need to remember that they are *always* role models and instruments of institutional and systemic change. As change agents, counselors and educators also need to remind themselves constantly that the change process is evolutionary in nature—slow, prone to resistance upon the part of every person and facet of the established institution or system, negatively as well as positively shaped by the countertransference dynamics of each human being in the institution or system, and even affected by the "collective countertransference" of the organization. Counselors and educators need to expect institutions and systems to change, and they need to be *actively* committed to initiating and maintaining adaptive organizational methods for resolving or more effectively managing countertransference. These are *daily* goals and struggles that evolve into career-long objectives for those of us who persist in the chemical dependency treatment and education field (Adams, 2000).

Education is always key to the resolution and management of countertransference within the counselor-client relationship as well as within the context of systems and institutions. Counselors become educational agents of institutional countertransference resolution vis-à-vis the context of their effective and successful counseling relationships with chemically dependent or substance-abusing persons. The mere presence of a professional chemical dependency counselor or chemical dependency treatment unit in a hospital or an institution represents an ongoing potential source of various forms of countertransference resolution. Counselors and program administrators need to encourage the growth and development of educational activities that promote awareness and insight within institutions or systems.

The administrators and directors of institutions and systems should also be the focus of intensive and ongoing drug education efforts. The resolution of institutional and systemic countertransference begins at the top levels of management, rather than with custodial or food service personnel. Substance abuse and chemical dependency problems are not going to somehow magically disappear or go into remission throughout the various institutions in America and the world. Thus, all people composing an institution or system need to understand better the devastating effects of substance abuse and become motivated to work toward changing personal or systemic sources of countertransference associated with this reality.

Chemical dependency is an illness or disease that adversely impacts every human being in a plethora of costly and destructive ways. Collective and individual solutions to the various problems of substance abuse and chemical dependency do not evolve from the countertransference mechanisms of denial, minimization, avoidance, projection, prejudice, and rationalization. The resolution and management of institutional countertransference is but one of the major keys to the successful amelioration of individual and collective chemical dependency problems.

SUMMARY

Countertransference is a fundamental component in all counseling and psychotherapy relationships, impacting the counseling relationship in a diversity of destructive as well as potentially constructive ways. This chapter examined a number of methods for resolving and managing the destructive or psychonoxious countertransference reactions that occur in counselor-client relationships as well as in institutions and systems.

Counselor selection methods can be utilized to reduce countertransference problems. Chemical dependency counselor selection characteristics were outlined in this chapter.

The education and clinical training of professional chemical dependency counselors constitutes another method for reducing countertransference distortion in counselor-client relationships and in institutions. Counselor education and training experiences foster trainee understanding, insight and awareness, and skill building that can help avoid countertransference distortion in clinical practice and institutional settings. Basic guidelines for the didactic course work and clinical training requirements for professional chemical dependency counselors were outlined in this chapter. Counselor selection, education, and training need to be conceptualized as ongoing processes.

Counselor supervision represents perhaps the single most effective method for resolving and managing countertransference. Supervision is an extension of the process of counselor selection, education, and training. Suggestions were provided in this chapter relative to the intensity and structure of the supervisory relationship. Behavioral science education (counselor education, psychology, psychiatry, social work, etc.) and training programs need to employee faculty and staff members who are experienced, well-trained, and skilled in the areas of chemical dependency supervision, treatment, training, and assessment. Chemical dependency counselors should be involved in some form of supervisory relationship for the duration of their clinical work (Culbreth and Borders, 1999).

Counselor trainees and even practicing therapists are sometimes required to enter personal therapy or analysis in order to resolve countertransference conflicts and other personal problems. Many graduate programs require students to undergo personal counseling or psychotherapy in order to fulfill graduation requirements (Aspy et al., 2000). Psychoanalysts are required to complete several hundred hours of personal psychoanalysis to be certified to practice in the field. Personal therapy can be viewed as a rather logical extension of the counselor selection, education, training, and supervision processes. However, personal therapy provides a significantly more extensive, in-depth, focused, and resolution-oriented method for ameliorating countertransference distortion.

The dynamics of as well as potential methods for resolving and managing institutional and systemic countertransference were also discussed in this chapter. Countertransference reactions to chemical dependency occur in institutions and all systems as well as within the context of counselor-client relationships. The education and training of top-level administrators in organizations is key to the resolution and management of institutional and systemic countertransference reactions related to substance abuse and chemical dependency (Adams, 2000).

Chapter 6

Therapeutic Dimensions of Countertransference

INTRODUCTION

As indicated in earlier chapters, countertransference has histori-cally been viewed as a major source of the negative or potentially unhealthy components of therapist behavior and response within the context of the therapeutic relationship. Recent characteriza-tions of countertransference phenomena in chemical dependency counseling emphasize the ambivalence associated within this con-struct (Shaffer, 1994; Forrest, 1998a; Carruth, 2000). However, Schultz and Hughes (1995) indicate that nearly all psychoanalytic schools now acknowledge the constructive and useful aspects of countertransference.

This chapter examines the healthy and constructive therapeutic dimensions of countertransference in chemical dependency coun-seling. Many analysts and dynamically oriented therapists have long emphasized that countertransference can facilitate growth, personality change, and enhanced self-awareness upon the part of the client as well as the therapist. The various roles of counter-transference in the process of facilitating adaptive client change are elucidated in this chapter, including the therapeutic dimen-sions of countertransference-related empathy; human attachment and relatedness; the countertransference-transference matrix; thera-pist disclosure of countertransference; countertransference in re-lapse prevention and treatment termination; countertransference and the diagnostic process; and counselor self-awareness, educa-tion, and growth.

COUNTERTRANSFERENCE, EMPATHY, AND THE CAPACITY FOR HUMAN ATTACHMENT AND RELATEDNESS

Ferenczi (1950/1919), Reik (1948), and Sullivan (1953) emphasized that the analyst or counselor is a "human being." Reik (1948) states:

> The psychoanalyst is a human being like any other, and not a god. There is nothing superhuman about him. In fact, he has to be human. How else could he understand other human beings? If he were cold and unfeeling, a "stuffed shirt" as some plays portray him, he would be an analytic robot or a pompous, dignified ass who could not gain entry to the secrets of the human soul. (p. 154)

Countertransference is a basic manifestation of the therapist's capacity to empathize with the client. The countertransference reactions of the counselor are also manifestations of his or her humanness and capacities for human attachment and relatedness. In the absence of healthy and appropriate countertransference reactions, the counselor's ability to empathize with the client and to form a working and productive therapeutic alliance is limited or flawed. The therapist and client must both manifest the capacities for human attachment, bonding, and relatedness in order to develop a working and productive therapeutic relationship.

Empathy (Shaffer, 1994) has been defined as "the inner experience of sharing in and comprehending the momentary psychological state of another person" (p. 345). Empathy also includes vicarious introspection and emotionally knowing another person. Tansey and Burke (1989) indicate that the empathic experience is characterized in the therapist by feelings of "harmony and closeness with the patient," as well as by the experience of "positive self-regard for performing a job well" (p. 41). The author (Forrest, 1992) has indicated that empathy is an essential ingredient in successful psychotherapeutic encounters and defines accurate empathy as "the ability of the therapist to be both affectively and cognitively attuned to what the patient is currently feeling and experiencing and to communicate to the patient an understanding of these feelings" (p. 10).

The cold, aloof, detached, and countertransference*less* therapist fails to communicate overtly to the client his or her ability to "feel with" the client. Therapists who are devoid of healthy countertransference reactions find it extremely difficult, if not impossible, to understand and empathize with the feelings, cognitions, and behaviors of their clients. They are unable to comprehend the internal world of their clients or therapeutically experience their clients' internal frame of reference.

Countertransference reactions also influence and encompass the therapist's capacity for experiencing and expressing nonpossessive warmth for the client. Nonpossessive warmth is an essential ingredient in effective psychotherapy relationships and refers to

> the therapist's warm acceptance of the patient (both experiences and feelings) without any conditions. The therapist accepts what is, rather than being concerned with what should be . . . warmth is a precondition for the therapist to accurately perceive the inner feelings and experiences of the patient, as well as a precondition for the patient's trust and self-exploration. (Forrest, 1992, p. 10)

Thus, the counselor's capacity for healthy countertransference impacts his or her ability to empathize with the client and demonstrate nonpossessive warmth toward the client within the therapeutic encounter. These countertransference-related counselor skills also facilitate the development of client trust and more in-depth self-exploration in therapy. These factors further reinforce the development of therapeutic bonding, or attachment, intimacy, and healthy human relatedness within the therapeutic relationship.

The healthy countertransference reactions of the therapist are an expression of therapist genuineness or authenticity. The author (Forrest, 1992) indicates that

> with regard to the essential ingredients of successful therapy, therapist genuineness or authenticity is the most fundamental . . . genuineness is defined as the therapist's ability to be open

to his own experience within the therapeutic encounter and to honestly express these feelings to the patient. More simply, the therapist is a real person; he or she wears no façade, expresses feelings and experiences to the patient within the therapeutic encounter, and makes every effort to relate in a personally relevant manner within this context. (p. 9)

To a varying degree, the therapist's genuineness or self-disclosing behavior is always an expression of his or her countertransference and basic humanness within the context of the therapeutic relationship.

The client's experience of the counselor or therapist as a "real person" within the therapeutic encounter can be a reinforcer and catalyst for further openness, self-disclosure, empathy, and reflective warmth upon the part of the client. The healthy countertransference-oriented reactions and responses of the counselor thereby reinforce and encourage the client's expression of basic humanness and authenticity within the therapeutic relationship. This process subsequently strengthens the therapeutic alliance and fosters the progressive development of more depth, intimacy, meaning, and attachment in the relationship between the counselor and client (Hill, 2000).

It is apparent that the countertransferential reactions of the counselor are a vehicle for counselor-client attachment, bonding, relatedness, and interaction in the therapeutic dyad. Reik (1948) alluded to the reality of the therapist being a robotic automaton in the absence of various countertransference phenomena in the psychotherapy relationship. He was astutely correct in this observation! The core therapeutic qualities of the counselor (Aspy et al., 2000) are included in the countertransference, and it is essential that these qualities or conditions be communicated to the client and understood by the client.

THE COUNTERTRANSFERENCE-TRANSFERENCE MATRIX

As touched upon briefly in the introduction to this text, countertransference reactions and/or distortions always occur in response to and/or are related to the transference reactions of the client. Transference refers to the *patient's* distorted or neurotic responses to the psychotherapist and the psychotherapy relationship (Forrest, 1999). Transference evolves from the patient's parataxic early life experiences and emotions that stem from parental and familial interactions. Within the context of the therapeutic relationship, the patient begins to relate to the therapist as a father figure, an extension of the mother-object, or a significant other. In sum, the client projects or "transfers" his or her various conflicts of the past onto the therapist. Transference reveals many of the client's most basic conflicts and problems. Resolution of the client's transference neurosis is believed to be tantamount to a successful psychoanalytic treatment outcome.

Slakter (1987) indicates that countertransference consists of "the analyst's reactions to the patient's transference, to the material the patient brings in, and to the patient's response to him as a person" (p. 24). This author also believes that since countertransference is basically induced by the patient's transference, personality, and behavior, it therefore provides the therapist with vital information about the patient. Countertransference is a tool for therapist self-understanding as well as understanding of the patient.

The client's transference reactions to the counselor and the counseling relationship may invoke powerful and intense countertransference in the counselor. However, the counselor's countertransference reactions to the client may also be bland or rather placid during various junctures in the therapeutic process. Nonetheless, *all* of the countertransference-oriented behaviors, cognitions, affects, and interactions between the counselor and client provide ongoing opportunities for the counselor as well as the client to learn, grow, and change. The countertransference-transference matrix also continually affects the therapeutic alliance (Neumann and Gamble, 1995) and always provides the opportunity for potentially constructive personality growth and change to occur within the context of the therapeutic relationship. Thus, constructive individual as well as mutual or relationship change and growth potentially evolve as a function of the countertransference-transference matrix.

Therapists learn about themselves and become more sensitive and self-aware as a function of client transference. Countertransference also fosters self-awareness in the counselor and simultaneously enhances the counselor's insight and awareness into the client's psychological being. The counselor can enhance the client's self-awareness and potential for constructive change and growth by (1) helping the client explore his or her transference reactions; (2) becoming more consciously aware of the various dynamics of his or her countertransference reactions and understanding how countertransference impacts self, the client, and the therapeutic relationship; and (3) openly sharing and integrating appropriate countertransference material at the appropriate times with the client. In essence, both the therapist and the client can learn and grow via the process of dealing with transference and countertransference issues in the therapeutic relationship. The countertransference-transference matrix provides both the counselor and the client with a multifaceted relational learning environment.

It is of paramount importance that the counselor consciously understand and be able to accurately identify countertransference and transference material in the psychotherapy relationship. The therapeutic efficacy of the counselor is limited by the parameters of his or her ability to manage globally the various realities and vicissitudes of countertransference and transference within the ongoing context of the therapeutic alliance. A consistent, keen sensitivity to the various nuances of the countertransference-transference matrix enables the counselor to understand better various aspects of self, the client, and the therapeutic relationship.

THERAPIST DISCLOSURE
OF COUNTERTRANSFERENCE

Orthodox psychoanalysts and traditional psychoanalytically oriented psychotherapists have been trained to strictly avoid the disclosure of countertransference material to patients. However, contemporary counselors and therapists are generally far more prone to disclosing their countertransference reactions to clients. Maroda (1994) states that the general rule of thumb or underlying principle of *when* to disclose and analyze the countertransference is simple:

"The patient will simply tell you." Patients will either directly or indirectly request disclosure of countertransference material. For example, the patient might ask the therapist, "Are you angry with me?" or "Do I make you uncomfortable?" Indirect requests for countertransference disclosure often evolve vis-à-vis the patient's use of projective identification. Projective identification can be thought of as "the unconscious mind of the patient attempting to communicate to the therapist that which is unavailable consciously. For example, the patient whines and criticizes his therapist endlessly for not being loved enough. The disavowed affect is hate, which is stimulated in the therapist" (Maroda, 1994, p. 116). It may be more difficult for the therapist to recognize indirect patient requests for countertransference disclosure, and the therapist will generally be more ambivalent about these disclosures.

The counselor will always need to ask himself or herself many questions prior to openly disclosing countertransferential material to a client. It is essential that the counselor be comfortable with the countertransference before openly sharing it with the client. In general, if the therapist or counselor experiences significant discomfort regarding disclosure of the countertransference, then he or she should not share the material with the client at that time. It may be more appropriate and therapeutically efficacious to disclose particular countertransference material later or at several other junctures in the therapeutic process.

Interestingly, Maroda (1994) indicates that "the cardinal rule of (countertransference) disclosure is: Never tell the patient more than he wants to hear. And never assume that you know what that is. Always let him tell you" (p. 128). However, chemical dependency counselors are continually confronted with the paradoxical reality that their clients rarely, if ever, want to "hear" that they are chemically dependent. This is especially true during the initial stages of intensive therapy with substance abusers and/or addicted clients (Forrest, 1997b, 1999). Substance abusers, addicts, and clients with impulse control, antisocial, or passive-aggressive disorders (Forrest, 2000) are particularly prone to denying, minimizing, avoiding, repressing, projecting, distorting, and, in various other ways, simply not acknowledging and accepting responsibility for a plethora of their behaviors. As such, many of these clients are confused about what they want to "hear" or what they "have heard," and they may never honestly tell the counselor what it is they want or need to hear.

In view of these realities, it is essential that chemical dependency counselors be able to share openly some countertransference material with their clients during initial therapy sessions as well as throughout the course of therapy. For example, the counselor will need to express openly his or her concerns and sentiments about a client coming in for a counseling session while under the influence of alcohol or another mood-altering substance. Chemical dependency counselors need to address a diversity of issues associated with client relapse throughout the therapeutic process. Substance abusers and addicts are notorious for failing to keep appointments, refusing to pay bills, terminating prematurely, verbally attacking counselors, and refusing to take medications or follow the counselor's recommendations (Bratter and Forrest, 1985; Forrest, 1998a). In all of these situations, counselors will experience countertransference reactions, and they will need to disclose and discuss some or many facets of this countertransference with clients.

The appropriate disclosure of countertransference reactions by the chemical dependency counselor constitutes a method whereby the counselor *confronts* the clients with the various realities of their substance abuse, irresponsible behavior, narcissism, and so forth (Forrest, 1992). The therapeutic sharing of countertransference material by the counselor provides direct feedback to the client and may help effect thinking changes, behavioral change, affective regulation, and enhanced interpersonal functioning upon the part of the client. The adaptive countertransferential feedback and disclosures of the counselor may be incorporated and introjected by the client, thus potentially affecting global personality growth and change. The therapeutic gains associated with disclosing countertransference material are sometimes evident early in the treatment process; however, these gains become increasingly salient and powerful during the middle and later stages (Forrest, 1999) of the psychotherapeutic process.

Research (Jourard, 1964; Forrest, 1970; Hountras and Forrest, 1970; Forrest, 1978, 1997b) consistently indicates that there are optimal and therapeutically beneficial levels of counselor self-disclosure in therapy relationships as well as unhealthy or psychonoxious levels of counselor self-disclosure. Likewise, countertransference disclosure can impact the therapeutic relationship, the client, and the counselor in a diversity of constructive, destructive, or neutral ways. Premature, overdetermined, repetitive, and affectively charged countertransference disclosures are usually reflective of true countertransference distortions and often negatively impact the client, the therapeutic relationship, and eventually the therapist.

As noted in earlier chapters, chemical dependency counselors who are themselves recovering from addiction may be especially at risk for experiencing countertransference distortion conflicts in their counseling relationships. Although it may be easier for the recovering counselor to empathize with the client and establish initial therapeutic rapport (Culbreth and Borders, 1999), many recovering counselors project their personal recovery and substance abuse histories onto the client, and their counseling sessions may consequently take the form of mutually sharing "drunk-a-logs." The counselor may actually harm the client and/or limit the effectiveness of the counseling relationship by flooding the client with countertransference-oriented disclosures. These counselor-client transactions are pathologically based upon the mutual medium of projective identification. The counselor may repetitively disclose many of the facets of his or her life, substance abuse history, and recovery process and believe, and indeed consciously attempt to teach the client, that there is only one royal road to recovery and change—the counselor's road! Obviously, these transactions are limited and generally unhealthy.

With these various pitfalls in mind, it is true that the recovering chemical dependency counselor may possess certain therapeutic advantages and skills that the nonrecovering clinician does not have. The recovering counselor does share common experiential material, serves as a concrete/living role model, and can actively and deeply empathize with the substance-abusing or chemically dependent client. When recovering counselors are able to consistently and appropriately control their countertransference disclosures throughout the course of therapy, they can be very successful in their treatment relationships with this patient population.

Healthy counselor countertransference disclosures can be used as a tool for teaching the client about feelings, relationships, substance abuse, and addiction; paths to recovery and change; relapse, awareness and self-dialogue; and a plethora of other important issues pertaining to human interactions and the nature of effective living (Hill, 2000).

COUNTERTRANSFERENCE IN RELAPSE PREVENTION AND TREATMENT TERMINATION

The therapist's awareness of client resistance, addictive patterns of thinking, and relapse dynamics can be utilized as deterrents to client relapse. For example, the author recently found himself feeling concerned with and somewhat preoccupied about a client who had remained totally alcohol/drug abstinent throughout the course of some sixteen months of individual and group psychotherapy. This client was in the process of terminating therapy and was being seen only in individual therapy once a month. The client had dropped out of a recovery support group over a period of six months in spite of active encouragement by the author for him to remain engaged with this group. The author dreamed that he was stopped in his car by a police officer (the client was, in fact, a police officer!), and the officer in this dream was obviously acutely intoxicated. When the author shared this dream with his recovering client a few weeks later, the client admitted that he had recently been consciously thinking a great deal about "using" and was struggling with several relapse-oriented issues. He decided to return to the support group, reengaged in individual therapy every other week for two months, and did not experience a relapse.

This is an excellent example of the therapeutic utilization of countertransference as a deterrent to relapse during the termination phase of intensive chemical dependency therapy. The counselor's sensitivity to self-oriented as well as client-oriented feelings of anxiety, interpersonal conflict, anger, depression, drug craving, self-defeating behaviors, and other psychodynamics can become manifest in the countertransference. The disclosure and exploration of such countertransference material can help deter the process of relapse in substance-abusing or chemically dependent persons. In such cases, the preconscious or unconscious awareness of the counselor is in touch with the preconscious or unconscious being of the client, and this material becomes real and accessible to conscious expression via the countertransference. Efficacious counselor management of countertransference can deter the relapse process. Counselor insensitivity, lack of self-awareness, and an inability to control or manage countertransference distortion can facilitate and destructively synergize the relapse process.

The process of termination in intensive chemical dependency counseling can be difficult for both the client and the counselor (Forrest, 1997b, 1998a, 1999). Indeed, the termination stage of intensive chemical dependency counseling may be emotionally stressful for the counselor, provoking significant countertransference. The termination process in intensive chemical dependency counseling usually evokes significant feelings of loss, grief, mourning, and separation in the counselor and the client. Clients are also prone to experiencing transference conflicts associated with feelings of abandonment, anxiety, and rejection. Many chemical dependency counselors experience neurotic struggles related to "letting go" of their clients during the termination phase of therapy (Forrest, 1997b). Relationship symbiosis and dependency issues may impact both counselor and client during this stage of the therapeutic process.

These various sources of countertransference teach and educate the counselor about his or her personal struggles and feelings associated with the termination process, and this simultaneously makes the counselor much more aware and sensitive to the client's feelings, reactions, and cognitions related to termination. Countertransference problems can lead to premature therapy terminations, protracted terminations, and lackluster endings to the process of counseling. Countertransference must be explored and integrated into the termination process in order to effect an optimally successful treatment termination. Indeed, countertransference is a significant component of the process of terminating a counseling or psychotherapy relationship.

Little has been written about the process of termination in chemical dependency counseling (Forrest, 1997b), or about the consistent impact of the termination process upon the psyche of the therapist. Klauber (1986) noted:

> It is strange that there seems to be no discussion of the effects on the analyst of forming relationship after relationship of the deepest and most intimate kind with patient after patient, and mourning which at some level must be involved for each of them." (p. 202)

It is important to note that intensive psychotherapy and counseling relationships consistently impact both the clinician and the client, as does the process of terminating these relationships.

Elsewhere (Forrest, 1991, 1999), I have indicated that many chemically dependent clients have never before experienced a consistently nurturing, intimate, supportive, loving, and healthy human relationship. These realities make it easier to understand and anticipate the manifestation of intense transference reactions associated with ending an intensive counseling relationship. As counselors and therapists, we tend to deny, scotomize, and minimize our own reactions, humanness, and countertransference associated with terminating treatment relationships. Perhaps we expect ourselves, and our clients also expect us, to be generally devoid of strong feelings and thoughts in response to treatment terminations. In reality, counselors do experience countertransference during the termination stage of therapy, and this countertransference is (1) a normal component of the termination process and (2) a viable and healthy teaching, education, and awareness-building medium for self, the client, and the therapeutic relationship.

Although the counselor may have been fortunate enough in the process of life and daily living to have experienced several loving, nurturing, and intimate human relationships, he or she is nonetheless subject to the internal experience of grief, loss, mourning, and various other strong effects in response to termination. Termination-centered countertransference may also stimulate a personal sense of success, professional and personal satisfaction and accomplishment, happiness, envy, and excitement in the counselor. However, Klauber (1986) astutely emphasized that the counselor experiences countertransference repetitively for the duration of his or her practice as a result of "forming relationship after relationship of the deepest and most intimate kind with patient after patient" (p. 116). Indeed, termination-centered countertransference can be viewed as a repetition-compulsion component of the process of all forms of intensive psychotherapy. This process can be stimulating and growth enhancing for the counselor as well as stressful and perhaps emotionally damaging over the course of twenty to forty years.

COUNTERTRANSFERENCE AND THE DIAGNOSTIC PROCESS

Countertransference can be a useful clinical tool in the counselor's diagnostic armamentarium. Searles (1987) has found that "the countertransference gives one one's most reliable approach to the understanding of patients of whatever diagnosis . . . the diagnosis should begin with the study of the interviewer's own emotional reactions to the interactions between the patient and himself" (p. 131). The counselor's various countertransference reactions can be utilized clinically to assess and diagnose the client throughout the course of treatment. Countertransference can aid the processes of initial diagnosis, differential diagnosis, and the assessment of client change and growth in therapy.

Diagnosis is process oriented. The diagnostic process begins when the counselor initially meets the client, invoking the counselor's initial countertransference reactions. Ongoing counselor-client interactions continuously involve assessment (Knauert, 2000) and the countertransference of the counselor. Once a clinician has formulated an initial diagnostic impression of the client, this formulation is openly and honestly shared with the client (Forrest, 1978, 1997b). This process is akin to openly sharing select countertransference material. Diagnostic impressions may also be shared and discussed openly throughout treatment. This technique fosters several sources of therapeutic gain:

1. It is reality oriented and based upon counselor openness and honesty rather than denial or distortion.
2. It helps define and maintain the counselor-client relationship.

3. It further assesses client motivation and readiness for therapy.
4. It may serve to instill a sense of hope and optimism in the client relative to seeking and remaining engaged in counseling, as diagnosis literally means "knowing through."

Thus, countertransference material may enhance the diagnostic process and the treatment outcome, as well as facilitate the process of establishing an appropriate treatment plan and identifying individualized treatment goals.

When the counselor openly and honestly shares his or her diagnostic impression with the client, he or she enlists the magic of words and communicates to the client, "Your problem is known and has causes. We can work together to effect constructive and positive change." This technique can be tremendously therapeutic for many chemically dependent or substance-abusing persons. In part, this therapeutic technique utilizes the countertransference to help the client better accept the reality of his or her addictive self and also confronts a variety of issues associated with the basic stigmas, labels, and behaviors that are central to recovery and the additive process (Forrest, 1998a; 1999).

As touched upon earlier, countertransference distortions and conflicts tend to be more intense and frequent when the chemically dependent client manifests concurrent or comorbid major mental illness, severe personality disorder, bipolar illness, or neurologic impairment. Many schizophrenic and acutely psychotic persons are also alcohol dependent or abuse various psychoactive substances (Bellack, 2000). These clients trigger or exacerbate counselor countertransference distortions involving feelings of intense anxiety, confusion, fragmentation, and ego defusion. Antisocial substance abusers and addicts often precipitate countertransference reactions involving feelings of fear, anxiety, threat, anger, and inadequacy in many counselors (Forrest, 1996). The chemically dependent client with a comorbid borderline personality disorder may trigger intense feelings of anxiety in many chemical dependency counselors. These clients tend to make their counselors feel "crazy" at various junctures in the therapeutic process. Substance abusers and chemically dependent clients who manifest bipolar illness or a severe affective disorder may trigger countertransference reactions in counselors that are associated with depressive affect, agitation, or a personal sense of hopelessness. Heroin addicts, polydrug dependents, brain-damaged persons, and other client subpopulations may trigger a diversity of intense and conflicted countertransference reactions in chemical dependency counselors (Hahn, 2000).

An accurate diagnosis or differential diagnosis (Knauert, 2000) of the chemically dependent client's co-occurring psychiatric disorder facilitates more effective treatment outcomes as well as the containment or amelioration of many sources of counselor countertransference distortion. Thus, it is essential that the chemical dependency counselor be able to diagnose and assess accurately both substance use disorders as well as various psychological/psychiatric disorders and either provide various appropriate individualized treatment interventions or refer clients for appropriate individualized care (Bellack, 2000; Heil, Wong, and Higgins, 2000).

Chemically dependent or substance-abusing persons with co-occurring severe psychiatric illness almost always precipitate more intense, pathologic, and personally disturbing countertransference reactions in chemical dependency counselors and other mental health workers. Therefore, it is essential that counselors and staff who work with these very difficult patient subpopulations employ the various methods and strategies that are elucidated throughout this text to reduce or minimize countertransference distortion and conflicts.

COUNTERTRANSFERENCE AND COUNSELOR SELF-AWARENESS, EDUCATION, AND GROWTH

As touched upon in earlier chapters, countertransference can be employed as a positive therapeutic instrument that fosters counselor or therapist self-awareness, education, and personal growth, as well as adaptively influencing the client and counselor-client relationship. A basic counselor dictum is simply, "Counselor, know thyself," and the process of evolving counselor self-awareness is always tied to the countertransference in therapeutic work. Self-awareness and self-understanding or self-education in psychotherapy occur vis-à-vis the counselor's cognitive, affective, and interpersonal interactions with the client. The counselor's sensitivity and general awareness of self, the client, and interactive relationship dynamics in the countertransference will ultimately foster or constrict his or her capacities for heightened self-awareness.

The counselor's reactions, feelings, and thoughts about his or her clients provide a valuable source of self-education. It is imperative that the counselor be consciously aware of his or her various reactions to the client and also be open to the process of self-experience in the therapeutic relationship in order to utilize the countertransference optimally in a therapeutically efficacious manner.

Many counselors attempt to deny, minimize, or repress their countertransference reactions. Counselor educators and supervisors frequently hear their supervisees and students report, "I'm not afraid of him," "I don't really hate Mr. X," "I can work with her," or "She doesn't push my buttons," when, in fact, trainees may be experiencing very profound and intense countertransference reactions (Celenza, 1995). Counselors and therapists are often afraid to acknowledge countertransference and irrationally believe they should either not experience these reactions or be able to manage the countertransference personally. An essential task of the supervising clinician is simply that of helping the counselor trainee become more aware of countertransference. Once this process begins in the supervisory relationship, the trainee can also become more open and disclosing about countertransference material, and, thus, trainee sensitivity and awareness are enhanced. The supervising clincian can also use trainee countertransference as a teaching and educational tool within the context of the supervisory relationship.

The process of effectively managing and dealing with countertransference material via the counselor education and training process as well as ongoing clinical practice is always educational, stimulating, and a resource for personal growth and constructive development upon the part of the counselor. Counselors and therapists can grow and become better or more effective clinicians and people as a result of recognizing, understanding, and dealing with countertransference.

Healthy counselor self-disclosure of countertransference material fosters client self-awareness and growth. The counselor, in effect, also educates or teaches the client about how the client is perceived by others (e.g., the counselor) and how others experience different thoughts, feelings, and reactions within the context of intimate human encounters. These processes occur via healthy counselor countertransference disclosures. The counselor models and may use direct educational and communication techniques to teach the client to better understand, recognize, express, and manage various facets of the self.

Just as countertransference material can be utilized to stimulate counselor self-awareness, education, and personal growth, so too can the countertransference be employed to stimulate the transference and transference-oriented self-other awareness, education, and growth in clients. Thus, countertransference can always provide a proven avenue to enhance counselor and client generalized interpersonal awareness, education, and growth, as well as the therapeutic alliance.

SUMMARY

Freud (1961/1912) alluded to the therapeutic utilization of the analyst's countertransference (unconscious) to understand the patient's unconscious:

> To put into a formula, [the analyst] must turn his own unconscious like a receptive organ toward the transmitting microphone. Just as the receiver converts back into soundwaves the electric oscillations . . . so the doctor's unconsciousness is able, from the derivatives of the unconscious which are communicated to him, to reconstruct the unconscious, which has determined the patient's free associations. (pp. 111-112)

Thus, Freud both understood and acknowledged the therapeutic uses of countertransference. Countertransference can be viewed as a component of the therapist's self-system that is utilized to comprehend or "read" the client.

Countertransference is a major component of the psychological process whereby the counselor is able to empathize and interact with the client in a manner that overtly, and at various levels of consciousness, communicates his or her basic humanness and capacities for human attachment and relatedness. Definitions of empathy are included in this chapter as well as the countertransference-related therapeutic characteristics of nonpossessive warmth and therapist genuineness or authenticity. It is imperative that the countertransference-related therapeutic characteristics of the counselor be communicated to the client and understood or perceived by the client.

Countertransference is always associated with transference phenomena in the context of intensive chemical dependency counseling (Forrest, 1997b). Thus, the countertransference-transference matrix continually evolves and affects the counselor, client, and counseling relationship throughout the course of treatment. A definition of transference is included in this chapter. The therapeutic aspects of the countertransference-transference matrix are also explored in this chapter.

The author generally advocates sharing countertransference material with clients, and guidelines for the therapeutic management of this complex and sometimes difficult therapeutic task are outlined. Maroda's (1994) cardinal rule of countertransference disclosure involves never telling the client "too much," never assuming that you (the counselor) know what "too much" is, and always letting the client tell you what he or she needs to hear. The risks and unhealthy aspects of countertransference disclosure are also discussed in this chapter.

Countertransference material can be used therapeutically to confront the client as well as to deter relapses and to resolve or more effectively manage the various issues associated with the process of terminating therapy. The countertransference can also be used as (1) a diagnostic tool, (2) a barometer of client change or index of ongoing treatment progress, and (3) a vehicle for enhancing counselor self-awareness and facilitating ongoing counselor personal growth and education.

In contrast to the viewpoints and interpretations of the early analysts, countertransference can be a wellspring of constructive growth and change in virtually all psychotherapy relationships. Chemical dependency counselors need to be very cognizant of the basic therapeutic dimensions of countertransference (Carruth, 2000) that were examined in this chapter.

Chapter 7

Countertransference Issues in the Twenty-First Century

INTRODUCTION

It is apparent that the concept of countertransference has evolved and changed significantly over the past one hundred years. The countertransference construct will continue to evolve and change as the behavioral science and health care professions move into the twenty-first century. While it is difficult to predict the evolution of the countertransference construct into the distant future, counselors and therapists continue to experience a multiplicity of here-and-now-oriented clinical realities associated with countertransference. As a result of this combination of historic and present understanding of countertransference in clinical practice, we are also better able to predict a number of general areas that will be particularly influenced by countertransference issues in the twenty-first century on a daily basis.

This chapter elucidates many important countertransference-related issues that are currently and may be futuristically associated with ethics, gender and multicultural realities, managed care, client comorbidity, and the dual-diagnosis client. Practicing chemical dependency counselors and other health care providers who work with substance abusers and chemically dependent persons as well as persons receiving mental health/psychiatric care have been forced to deal with these particular countertransference-related issues for a decade. These issues and other emergent clinical issues will continue to impact significantly chemical dependency counselors and the chemical dependency treatment field for many years to come, indeed, well into the twenty-first century.

ETHICS

Ethics generally refers to the science of moral values and duties or the study of the ideal human character, actions, and behavior. Ethical conduct also involves conforming to professional standards of conduct and behavior. The ethical codes of professions are based upon underlying ethical principles such as beneficence (doing good), nonmalfeasance (do no harm), autonomy, fidelity, and justice (Beauchamp and Childress, 1983).

As indicated by Dove (1995, 1997), the professional ethics of chemical dependency treatment "follows logically from the ethics which apply to health care in general, medicine, and mental health (1995, p. 21)." The chemical dependency treatment field has recently established minimum competency levels for professionals who work in this field. Training, education, and supervision standards have been developed at regional, state, and national levels to ensure quality of care to patients, third-party payers, and to maintain appropriate ethical standards of practice.

Countertransference issues impact every facet of ethical practice in the chemical dependency and mental health treatment fields. For example, therapist-client sexual involvements are *always* a result of severe therapist countertransference distortion. Clients are invariably harmed by sexual contact with counselors (Pope, 1986, 1991; Irons and Schneider, 1999), and this manifestation of countertransference distortion also frequently results in very significant adverse consequences for counselors (e.g., arrest, incarceration, lawsuits and malpractice litigation, loss of licensure, etc.). The actual countertransference dynamics may vary from counselor to counselor in situations involving counselor-client sexual contact, but in general the perpetrators in these cases manifest severe countertransference distortion related to power and control, poor impulse control, limit setting and boundary issues, trust, anger, psychopathy, gender and intimacy, and severe character pathology. The vast majority of therapist-client sexual relationships involve male therapists and female clients.

Countertransference is consistently related to a plethora of other ethical problems and dilemmas in the chemical dependency and mental health treatment fields. Insurance fraud, breech of confidentiality, self-referral practices, misrepresentation of treatment "success rates," "free initial evaluations," dual relationships, reimbursement policies, and "kickbacks" for referrals (Dove, 1995) are but a few of the thorny ethical dilemmas that have historically plagued the chemical dependency treatment field. These countertransference-driven sources of ethical misconduct have contributed to or directly resulted in public distrust of chemical dependency treatment programs and counselors; victimization of thousands of clients; closure of hundreds of residential treatment programs; the near collapse of the chemical dependency treatment field in the past eight years; and endless litigation, costs, and emotional damages for all who become involved in these tragic situations.

Dove (1995) states that "some of the unethical behaviors which have led to the present status [of the chemical dependency treatment field] could have been prevented with an appropriate training program in applied professional ethics" (p. 19). The author would stress the importance of training, education, supervision, and, in some cases, ongoing therapy or other measures dealing specifically with countertransference as a major component in all counselor/mental health worker training programs in applied professional ethics.

Chemical dependency counselors and all mental health workers will be required to better understand and maintain ethical standards of practice in the twenty-first century. Perhaps this increased awareness and demand for more ethical practice standards will also foster a keener and more sensitive appreciation of the many facets of countertransference in all helping relationships.

Kitchener (1986) has advocated the following goals for moral education:

1. Sensitize trainees to ethical issues.
2. Improve trainees' abilities to reason about ethical issues.
3. Develop moral responsibility and the ego-strength to take action.
4. Tolerate the ambiguity of ethical decision making.

Dove (1995) indicates that the goals for a continuing education program in applied professional ethics for chemical dependency workers should include the following:

1. increase staff sensitivity to ethical issues which arise in their day-to-day practice, 2. improve the ability of staff to reason about ethical dilemmas, 3. staff members should be able to formulate a plan of action based on the ethical analysis and follow through with the plan, and 4. improve coping mechanisms for tolerating the ambiguity of ethical decision making. (p. 28)

This author (Dove, 1997) has developed more specific and extensive suggestions for training chemical dependency counselors and staff.

It is significant that Dove (1995) indicates that

it is not enough for ethical codes to merely emphasize that any sexual contact between counselors and clients is a violation. Training must emphasize the harm done to clients, and the dynamic processes which underlie sexual interaction. This is often an uncomfortable area of discussion for supervisors as well as counselors. (p. 24)

Countertransference is at the heart of the "dynamic processes" that underlie sexual contact between chemical dependency counselors and clients and virtually every other form of unethical counselor behavior. As such, countertransference will continue to be a paramount issue in the realm of chemical dependency counselor ethics in the twenty-first century.

GENDER AND MULTICULTURAL REALITIES

The gender of the counselor impacts the client and the counseling relationship in myriad ways. Likewise, the gender of the client impacts the counselor, and gender-oriented issues always affect the therapeutic relationship in a multiplicity of ways. Countertransference dynamics are also always interactively affecting the gender-based realities of the client, counselor, and therapeutic dyad (Peterson, 2000).

Male counselors and therapists may interact and behave differently with male clients than they do with female clients. Counselor behaviors may also be influenced by the perceived physical attractiveness of clients, and this reality may be further affected by the gender combination of the therapeutic dyad. Some female clients feel uncomfortable or threatened by male therapists and will only engage in treatment with a female therapist. Other women are quick to seek out a male therapist and may even verbalize that they "don't like" or "don't trust" women in general. A few therapists (L. E. Wellman, personal communication, 1998) choose to limit their practices to same-gender clients.

Many heterosexual clients experience some level of anxiety or possibly feel threatened when their therapist is openly gay or lesbian. Homophobic clients might actively avoid any form of therapeutic relationship with counselors whom they perceive as homosexual or somehow sexually different. Openly gay or lesbian counselors can experience a diversity of uncomfortable feelings or thoughts in counseling relationships with bigoted or angry and threatening homophobic clients. The homosexual client will provoke anxiety, fear, or other countertransference reactions in many counselors. Countertransference issues are associated with the decision by some heterosexual counselors to avoid treating homosexual clients. Simply put, in any counseling relationship, the gender, sexual orientation, and global gender adjustment styles of the counselor-client dyad continually and significantly impact both the process and the outcome of treatment (Forrest, 1994; Holt, Houg, and Romano, 2000).

Transference and countertransference issues will continue to be associated with a diversity of counselor-client gender-based realities in the twenty-first century. Counselors as well as clients and the general public have become much more consciously aware of these realities over the past twenty years. It will be essential for counselors and clinicians of the twenty-first century to become increasingly sensitive, aware, and skilled in the therapeutic management of gender-based sources of countertransference and countertransference distortion.

Countertransference and transference processes are also related to ethnicity and a variety of multicultural realities. The general mental health needs of various racial and ethnic minority groups in the United States have not been adequately addressed (Greene,

1993; Okonji, Ososki, and Pulos, 1998; Garrett and Pichette, 2000). Counselor and client characteristics such as race and ethnicity have been related to the underuse of chemical dependency and/or mental health services by African Americans, Hispanics, Native Americans, and Asian Americans. Thompson, Worthington, and Atkinson (1994) report that African-American clients do not seek out mental health services, in part because African-American therapists are underrepresented in the counseling field. Research (Terrell and Terrell, 1984) also suggests that black clients experience greater mistrust and are more likely to terminate counseling when seen by a white counselor than when seen by a black counselor, and that black clients prefer to see a black counselor. Recent research evidence (Okonji, Ososki, and Pulos, 1998) seems to indicate that some ethnic minority clients tend to prefer directive approaches to counseling (reality therapy) over person-centered therapy. These issues are further complicated by the fact (Hill, 1998) that barely 5 percent of the membership of the American Psychological Association is composed of African Americans, Hispanics, Asians, and American Indians.

In clinical practice, countertransference and transference dynamics affect the counseling relationship in a number of ways. Many black, Hispanic, Native American, or other ethnic minority groups may prefer to work with counselors of the same or a similar ethnic background (Utsey et al., 2000). Some Caucasian clients will prefer to be seen by Caucasian counselors. Racial and ethnic realities may result in clients refusing to work with some counselors, and vice versa. Certainly, all counselors and therapists need to understand better the various influences and nuances of race, culture, gender, and social background and their effects on the process and outcome of chemical dependency counseling as well as mental health work in general (La Roche, 1999).

Countertransference phenomena can be extended to include multicultural issues that may be associated with religious background, socioeconomic class between and within various racial and ethnic groups, and ethnic value orientations. For example, the Irish Catholic male client might initially find it difficult to believe that he could be successfully treated for alcoholism, or even basically understood by a female Jewish counselor who has never consumed alcohol. Consider for a moment the possible multicultural realities that might come into play in the initial counseling session between an African-American male psychiatrist and a married, Caucasian, bisexual, chemically dependent, Italian mother of three children!

Counselors and therapists cannot realistically be expected to be equally therapeutic and effective in their relationships with all clients. Gender and multicultural issues (Peterson, 2000; Utsey et al., 2000) impact every counseling relationship, and this impact can have a "for better or worse" effect upon the process and outcome of therapy (Forrest, 1984, 1996). Multicultural issues (La Roche, 1999) also directly or more covertly influence the client's perceptions of the counselor and may impact virtually every facet of client behavior within the therapeutic relationship. These clinical realities often help to explain why a particular client may not become actively engaged in counseling or improve in treatment with one counselor but subsequently recover and improve dramatically while actively engaging in an ongoing working and highly productive therapeutic relationship with another counselor.

Chemical dependency counselors will need to be increasingly sensitive to the many countertransference-related multicultural issues that can potentially affect the counseling relationship in the twenty-first century. Awareness, understanding, sensitivity, education, training, and supervision will be the keys to the resolution of countertransference distortion that is related to multicultural factors. They will also facilitate counselor-client utilization of countertransference and transference processes to enhance the process and efficacy of psychotherapy in the future.

Counselor educators and all behavioral health educators need to be futuristically proactive in their efforts to educate, train, and employ chemical dependency counselors and mental health workers from a diversity of ethnic, racial, cultural, religious, and social groups.

MANAGED CARE

As every chemical dependency counselor and clinician in America has come to understand, managed care systems are really "managed cost" systems. The basic purpose of managed care is costcontainment (Howard and Mahoney, 1996; Strupp, 1997) or conserving health care monies. Strupp (1997) indicates that managed care is creating a reemergence of "the old two-tier system of medical care, that is, differential treatment of 'private patients' and 'clinic patients,' a disjunction between private care and indigent care, between 'first class' and 'economy class'" (p. 91).

Managed care has significantly impacted virtually all mental health and chemical dependency treatment personnel. The practical effects of managed care upon practicing counselors and clinicians include the following:

1. Briefer or limited therapy sessions
2. Significantly reduced fees and reimbursements for professional services
3. Increased paperwork and administrative demands upon providers
4. Increased competition between agencies and treatment providers for actual clients
5. Increased feelings of uncertainty and anxiety, confusion, and misunderstanding in many direct service providers as well as clients

A growing number of counselors and clinicians are choosing not to be involved in managed care. Health service providers are paying increasing attention to the ethical parameters (Dove, 1995, 1997; Walsh, 1998; Knapp and VandeCreek, 2000) of relationships between managed care systems, chemical dependency counselors, and all mental health workers and programs.

It is significant that many managed care organizations have eliminated or greatly reduced the number of psychiatrists and doctoral-level psychologists from their provider panels or lists. Master's-level clinicians are employed to provide individual therapy, marital therapy, chemical dependency counseling, consultation and evaluation or testing services, and various other mental health/ chemical dependency services. These individuals are frequently willing to provide professional services for $25 to $75 per session, while doctoral-level clinicians either charge substantially more for their services or are unwilling to work for significantly reduced fees. Apparently, some managed care systems attempt to reduce the need for actual counseling and direct clinical services by utilizing psychiatrists to prescribe a variety of psychotropic medications for clients who seek mental health and/or chemical dependency services. A plethora of ethical, quality of care, and other practical matters are associated with these managed care dilemmas.

As citizens and taxpayers, most Americans recognize the need for some system to accomplish the task of managing the costs of health care (mental health and chemical dependency services in the current context) in a manner that is fair and causes minimal hardships on consumers, professionals, and the public purse. This author would argue that such a system did not exist in the American health care arena in the 1980s, and as a result, (1) health care expenditures for mental health and chemical dependency services spiraled out of control, and (2) the "managed care era," in part, evolved in response to the overexpenditures, misexpenditures, and all too frequently unscrupulous and unethical billing procedures of mental health and chemical dependency providers of the 1980s.

It is readily apparent that countertransference issues played a significant role in the evolution of managed care in America. Countertransference dynamics and reactions overtly plague many chemical dependency counselors and mental health workers in their contemporary relationships with managed care and managed care clients. One might jokingly hypothesize that managed care systems will eventually eliminate all the vicissitudes of countertransference as well as transference in counseling and psychotherapy. After all, it is possible that the parameters of brief counseling and brief therapy in the futuristic world of managed care may evolve to the point of eliminating the development of a basic therapeutic relationship, thereby also eliminating countertransference and transference!

This author does not see such an evolution in the process of counseling taking place during the early twenty-first century, in spite of the best or worst efforts of our managed care systems. To the contrary, counselors and clinicians will struggle with even more intense and conflicted countertransference reactions associated specifically with managed care. Counselors will continue to struggle with countertransference based upon feelings of anger, anxiety, fear, insecurity, and confusion as they deal with managed care systems and clients in the next several years. Quality of care, confidentiality, access to care, provider competence, and other ethical matters (Walsh, 1998; Knapp and VandeCreek, 2000) continue to reinforce and stoke the countertransference-transference matrix of the twenty-first century.

The hope of the future rests with the reality that our health care systems in America and throughout the world are not static in nature. Thus, as managed care systems continue to evolve and change, we can hope that systemic as well as individual sources of countertransference distortion and transference conflict will be minimized and/or become less pathologic and conflictual as a result of these ongoing change processes.

CLIENT COMORBIDITY AND DUAL DIAGNOSIS

Many counselors and clinicians in the chemical dependency treatment field (Knauert, 1979, 2000; Forrest, 1994, 1996, 1999, 2000, 2001) have reported for decades that the vast majority of substance-abusing and/or chemically dependent clients who enter various treatment programs and facilities manifest a diversity of coexisting psychological or psychiatric problems. The concept of the "dual diagnosis" was coined within the chemical dependency treatment field some ten years ago, and this term was originally applied to clients who clearly manifested a severe substance use disorder in combination with a severe concurrent psychiatric illness such as schizophrenia, bipolar illness, or a personality disorder.

During the past few years, the term "comorbidity" (Irons, 1998) has either replaced or been used synonymously with the concept of "dual diagnosis," and both concepts continue to refer to persons who manifest a substance use disorder with concurrent psychiatric illness. This general client population was previously referred to as "secondary" alcoholics or substance abusers (Forrest, 1997b).

Clinicians from a diversity of settings report that they are experiencing an upsurge of comorbid or dual-diagnosis clients (Kuhn,

1998). Recent research in the mental health and chemical dependency treatment field (Helzer and Pryzbeck, 1988; Hesselbrock, Meyer, and Kenner, 1985; Rounsaville et al., 1983; Nace, 1990; Forrest, 1996, 2000) indicates that 15 to 65 percent of male alcoholics and narcotic addicts manifest a concurrent antisocial personality disorder. Borderline personality disorder is most likely the second most common personality disorder found in substance-abusing clients. As Nace (1990) states, "It would seem safe to assume from the clinical studies now available that within the substance-abusing population, the prevalence of personality disorder is at least 50%" (p. 187). Similar research evidence (Forrest, 1997a; Bellack, 2000) demonstrates the presence of comorbidity in 20 to 70 percent of individuals with schizophrenia, bipolar illness, depressive illness, and anxiety and panic disorders. In fact, it is realistic to expect that a substance use disorder will coexist with virtually all varieties of psychopathology or DSM-IV subgroups in 20 to 70 percent of cases.

Regardless of the variables associated with the increase in persons entering counseling, treatment facilities, and various forms of health care as a result of a dual diagnosis or multiple problems, it is simply axiomatic that the more disturbed and conflicted the client, the greater the probability that the counselor will manifest both countertransference and countertransference distortion. Thus, enhanced counselor awareness of the various complexities associated with treating dual-diagnosis clients may be expected to generate a continued appreciation for countertransference issues in the twenty-first century.

The countertransference-oriented realities that pertain to working with dual-diagnosis clients in hospitals, residential psychiatric and chemical dependency treatment programs, prisons and correctional environments (Forrest, 2000), and other institutional settings will persist and escalate in the twenty-first century. Clinicians (Curton and Parker, 1998) report that "dual-diagnosis programs" often contribute to the manifestation of counselor stress as well as staff burnout. In our attempts to better treat the growing population of dual-diagnosis clients, it is realistic to expect that more of these programs will be developed over the course of the next two decades.

Finally, the interactive realities and dynamics of ethics, gender and multicultural issues, economics, politics, managed care, and severity of client pathology can be expected to exacerbate counter-transference-oriented processes in all counselors and health service providers in the twenty-first century.

SUMMARY

This chapter provided a discussion of some of the most germane and important issues pertaining to countertransference in chemical dependency counseling as well as general mental health work in the twenty-first century: ethics, gender and multicultural realities, managed care, and difficult clients—persons who have recently been referred to by clinicians as comorbid or dually-diagnosed.

Countertransference is at the heart of every facet of counselor ethics and ethical practice. Ethics was defined in this chapter, and a brief history of the role and development of ethical standards within the chemical dependency treatment field was outlined. Countertransference distortion dynamics play a significant role in all cases involving counselor sexual abuse of clients and boundary violations (Irons and Schneider, 1999), breech of confidentiality, insurance fraud, and other forms of ethical misconduct. Several methods (Kitchener, 1986; Dove, 1995, 1997) for reducing or eliminating ethical misconduct and countertransference-related ethical violations upon the part of counselors and mental health workers in the twenty-first century were delineated in this chapter.

A multiplicity of gender and multicultural issues influences every facet of countertransference. The gender, sexual orientation and adjustment style, race and cultural background, and religious beliefs or socioeconomic background of the counselor and client affect each participant in the counseling relationship as well as the therapeutic dyad and the process and outcome of counseling. The arcane, surprising, most primitive, or most therapeutic aspects of countertransference and transference can be related to the gender and multicultural dimensions of the counselor-client dyad. The realities of being Irish, Catholic, black, Asian, male or female, heterosexual or bisexual, very affluent or homeless are but a few of the multicultural factors that facilitate or affect countertransference in chemical dependency counseling. Multicultural realities may even impact the client-counselor selection and preference process as well as treatment modality preferences (Okonji, Ososki, and Pulos, 1998; Hill, 1998; Peterson, 2000). These issues will continue to be relative to helping relationships in the twenty-first century.

Managed care will continue to evoke intense feelings, thoughts, and behavioral reactions in counselors as well as clients in the future. Some of the primary countertransference-oriented reactions of most mental health workers and chemical dependency counselors to the managed care movement have historically included anxiety, anger, mistrust, confusion, and ambivalence. Many health care providers seem to feel that managed care has eroded their ability to earn a living or function effectively and ethically (Knapp and VandeCreek, 2000) in the health care arena. Indeed, the managed care movement has stirred a variety of often intense and diverse countertransference reactions in chemical dependency counselors, and this process will continue. The managed care movement will not, paradoxically, eliminate countertransference and transference from the therapeutic process.

Chemical dependency counselors and mental health workers will also continue to be confronted with the various realities that are associated with treating increasingly difficult dual-diagnosis clients. These comorbid or dually diagnosed persons will comprise a growing segment of the treatment populations receiving care via community mental health centers, residential and outpatient chemical dependency treatment programs, county jails, state and federal correctional institutions, university and college counseling centers, and psychiatric hospitals as well as private practice. Counseling and treatment relationships with these difficult persons will continue to evoke countertransference in treatment providers of the twenty-first century.

Finally, it is apparent that ethics, gender and multicultural issues, managed care, and client comorbidity/dual diagnosis are all interactively associated with countertransference in chemical dependency counseling and mental health work *today,* and these interactive relationships will persist well into the twenty-first century.

Chapter 8

Summary

This text is about chemical dependency counseling and the chemical dependency counselor. More specifically, this book examines the vicissitudes of countertransference as it influences and impacts the counselor, client, counseling relationship, and process and outcome of chemical dependency counseling. This book is the first available in the chemical dependency treatment field and behavioral health/mental health arena to examine systematically and comprehensively the various complex parameters of countertransference in clinical work with chemically dependent and substance-abusing persons.

It is the author's opinion that countertransference contributes to treatment outcome failure and a diversity of other relational difficulties that consistently occur within the context of chemical dependency counseling and virtually all professional and systemic interactions with substance abusers and chemically dependent clients. Countertransference can also contribute to the successful psychotherapy and treatment of substance abusers and chemically dependent clients.

Following a general introduction in Chapter 1, definitional and historical perspectives of countertransference were provided in Chapter 2 of this book. Chapter 3 included an examination of countertransference in the specific realm of chemical dependency counseling. Countertransference distortion was defined and the primary sources of countertransference distortion in chemical dependency counseling were elucidated in Chapter 4. Techniques and strategies for resolving and managing countertransference and countertransference distortion in chemical dependency counseling were provided in Chapter 5. The constructive and therapeutic dimensions of countertransference in chemical dependency counseling were discussed in Chapter 6. Chapter 7 included a general discussion of contemporary and futuristic issues related to countertransference in chemical dependency counseling and clinical work: ethics, gender and multicultural realities, managed care, and client comorbidity/dual diagnosis. Countertransference issues will continue to impact clients, counselors, and counseling relationships in the foreseeable future.

As indicated in the Introduction, countertransference

1. reflects the unconscious and neurotic conflicts of the counselor or therapist, as well as his or her total being;
2. is usually related to the client's transference, personality, and adjustment style;
3. is an inevitable and even desirable component of the counseling or therapeutic relationship;
4. can potentially foster growth, education, and change upon the part of the counselor and client as well as within the context of the helping relationship; and
5. may destructively impact the counselor, client, and therapeutic relationship.

In essence, countertransference impacts and shapes every facet of counselor behavior and being within the context of the counseling relationship. Although many contemporary chemical dependency counselors and clinicians struggle with the Freudian and psychodynamic origins of the countertransference construct, all will ultimately agree that their personal (and often unconscious or preconsciously understood and recognized) feelings, beliefs, life experiences, values and cognitions, education and training experiences, and so forth affect their professional relationships and clinical work with these often difficult clients.

I would encourage chemical dependency counselors as well as all other behavioral health clinicians who provide direct clinical services for this patient population to more fully acknowledge, recognize, understand, examine, and therapeutically utilize their countertransference reactions. Clinical supervisors, counselor educators, and rehabilitation program managers and administrators also need to recognize more fully and rationally deal with the many nefarious issues that are related to countertransference.

Finally, it must be emphasized again that the numbers of substance-abusing and chemically dependent persons in America and throughout the world continue to grow exponentially. As indicated throughout this text, chemically dependent and substance-abusing persons tend to provoke intense countertransference reactions in the various persons, institutions, and organizations with whom they come into contact. Thus, police officers and law enforcement personnel, physicians, hospital emergency room staff, college and university faculty and administrators, employers, managers and coworkers, and family members and friends who are involved with chemically dependent and substance-abusing persons are subject to intense countertransference reactions in the course of their daily interactions with these individuals. Violence in the workplace, domestic and family violence, automobile accidents and accidents at home, health care costs, escalating adolescent suicide and violence, an exploding prison population (Forrest, 2000), unwanted pregnancies and sexual problems, psychiatric illness, poor academic performance and school problems, racial hatred and prejudice, and divorce and relational conflicts are but a few of our growing social realities that are either synergized or directly caused by substance abuse and chemical dependency. These growing social realities provoke a plethora of intense emotional reactions in every person, system, and institution in America. Countertransference is therefore a basic and universal component in all modes of human interaction.

This text will enhance the therapeutic skills and efficacy of chemical dependency counselors and substance abuse treatment personnel. The counselor or therapist's feelings of empathy, compassion, anger, frustration, despair, fear, anxiety, confusion, and, indeed, the total spectrum of other human feelings, cognitions, and behaviors that are associated with a client and/or the counseling relationship are manifestations of countertransference. The material presented in this text will help chemical dependency counselors and other treatment providers better recognize, understand, manage, and utilize countertransference therapeutically, effectively, and creatively within the context of their helping relationships.

Epilogue

Brief Personal Reflections on Countertransference

The completion of this text was a slow process and eventually required some five years. Yet, the actual writing, content, development, and subject matter of the book remained relatively easy and stimulating throughout the entire process.

I found myself continually reflecting upon my personal feelings, thoughts, and clinical experiences with many clients I had treated over the past twenty-five or thirty years as I worked to bring this book to fruition. These personal clinical experiences provided a wealth of countertransference-oriented material from which I was able to address the various topics presented throughout the book. All of this was relatively easy and personally non-threatening. My own countertransference reactions to hundreds, if not a few thousand, clients over the past thirty years had always been "manageable" and generally constructive. Many clients had stirred intense personal and situational countertransference reactions involving anxiety, fear, compassion, intimidation, anger, intense empathy, grave concern, warmth, love, hopelessness, and ambivalence. However, my own historic countertransference reactions had always been manageable, resolvable, and essentially nonthreatening to my ego integration and basic sense of psychological well-being.

Then one day in late October 1998, I received a summons through the mail indicating that I had been added to a lawsuit involving a former client whom I initially treated (two sessions) twenty years earlier. This suit had originally been filed some seven or eight years prior and was then refiled by a different attorney and now involved four defendants—including me. I was being sued for alleged professional malpractice! This was a new and devastating professional experience for me. I had been practicing as a doctoral-level licensed clinical psychologist for over twenty-eight years and had never before been sued or involved in any form of personal, professional legal matter. In all those years of practice, I had never even had a single grievance or complaint filed against me by a client or professional colleague!

The experience of being sued precipitated a diversity of intense and sometimes personally threatening feelings, cognitions, and reactions over a period of some sixteen months. I also suspect that I shall continue to reexperience and struggle with some of these intense reactions for many months, if not years or perhaps life. Following a sixteen-month period of "living with" the process of being sued for malpractice, and one month after being fully exonerated of this charge via a three-week jury trial, it seems in retrospect that this professional life experience has been both personally damaging and very destructive as well as painfully constructive. This experience did increase my awareness about the real risks and legal liabilities associated with being a therapist, but it also enhanced my general therapeutic sensitivity as well as my commitment to clients and the work of attempting to somehow make our community and world a better place. This experience also deeply reinforced my commitment to treating all human beings in a manner that enhances a basic sense of respect, dignity, equality, and self-worth.

It was very difficult to believe for several weeks that I was really being sued, but the eventual and ongoing experiences of meetings with my defense attorneys soon extinguished my denial about this painful and embarrassing reality. For the first time in my life, I began to experience protracted sleep disturbance and fatigue. Within a few months, my family and colleagues began to comment on my weight loss and they expressed concerns about my health. My thoughts and cognitions became increasingly obsessive-compulsive and focused around the various issues of "being sued." I feared losing my career and practice and I worried about the possibility of eventually not being able to support my family, pay bills, or provide for my children's educations. I became progressively less interested in sex, more self-absorbed, and less sensitive and interactive with my family. I became depressed and stressed and at times experienced intense feelings and fantasies of rage directed at my former client, the plaintiff, as well as at the plaintiff's attorney. It became crystal clear to me how so many people could distrust, dislike, disrespect, or even murder attorneys—especially "plaintiffs' attorneys."

Being sued was an extremely draining experience, both emotionally and physically. This experience damaged my family, children, extended family members, and friends as well as myself. This most painful and difficult personal experience, however, may have paradoxically benefited myself as well as my clients and many of the other people with whom I interact on a daily basis. Could the experience of being sued for professional malpractice possibly be a personal "growth experience"? If I can now and in the future answer yes to this question, my response surely must be skewed by the fact that I was eventually found to be not guilty of malpractice by every member of an eight-person jury following a three-week trial. How would I feel about the positive growth dimensions of this process had the jury verdict been guilty?

How did I ever survive the process of being sued for sixteen months? How did I survive a jury trial, 8:30 a.m. to 5:30 p.m., Tuesday through Friday, for *three* weeks? How was it possible to control or minimize the various sources of countertransference distortion that evolved during and as a result of this process?

On top of all this, my wife and I had learned three months before my trial that our youngest daughter, a senior in high school and president of her graduating class, needed heart surgery. Then, one day before my trial ended and before he could learn that I had been exonerated, my stepfather died. For several months, my mother and sister as well as my in-laws had been very upset about the emotional conflict and turmoil that the suit had created within our family system. The countertransference-oriented ramifications of my legal case were multifaceted and seemed to touch every facet of my life and being, yet I was able to survive this labyrinth of stress and emotional hell. But again, how was all this possible?

Several cognitive, behavioral, affective, physical, interpersonal, and spiritual resources and strengths helped me endure and eventually overcome this very stressful and evil process. These same resources and strengths were the keys to overcoming counter-transference distortions and continuing to function effectively as a therapist during this most difficult time.

The cognitive awareness and concomitant self-talk that goes with repeatedly recognizing and acknowledging that this professional crisis was very miniscule and insignificant in the grand scale of life were consistently helpful and therapeutic. This was certainly an upsetting and stressful life event, but it was not catastrophic. I was alive and healthy, continuing to practice and help clients on a limited basis; my family was healthy and intact; and in basically every other respect, my life remained unchanged! By cognitively focusing on these realities, I was able to continue the various daily and professional behaviors and behavior patterns that had always contributed to my well-being and general success in life.

The cognitive and behavioral commitments to continued physical exercise and good nutrition also played a tremendously important role in the process of effectively managing countertransference-oriented distortions in my life during these months. I continued to go to a health club and lift weights two to three times per week, and I kept walking and jogging five to six days of the week, and four to six miles per walk on the weekends. I continued to eat breakfast each morning as well as lunch and supper—as I had for all my life.

Perhaps the most debilitating component of this "survival process" involved sleep disturbance. From the beginning to the end of this experience, I experienced consistent difficulties with falling asleep and then awakening in the middle of the night, only to find myself obsessing and unable to go back to sleep. Finally, during the first week of my trial (following discussion with and at the suggestion of an office colleague), I contacted our family physician and obtained a prescription for Xanax and then actually used this medication for sleep purposes on three occasions during the trial. Within a few days after the trial, I was once again able to sleep soundly for six to seven hours each night, and I have not taken any form of medication for sleep since the trial.

Throughout the sixteen-month process of being sued, I was able to discuss consistently and openly my various feelings, thoughts, and reactions with my wife and children, an office colleague and psychologist of nearly twenty-five years, my attorney, and my secretary as well as my mother and sister. These daily interactions were cathartic, supportive, and emotionally and professionally lifesaving. Needless to say, my attorneys had instructed me to avoid discussing this matter with anyone other than my wife and a few others, such as my secretary, at the time that I initially made contact with them and my professional malpractice insurance provider. However, my attorneys as well as their office support staff quickly became another major source of support, guidance, education, and strength. At the end of the initial contact with my senior attorney, he actually encouraged me to call him if I needed "to talk" or for whatever other purposes and provided me with his home phone number. My St. Paul insurance carrier supervisor was equally understanding, supportive, and committed to my case. The attorneys who represented me in this case repeatedly encouraged me to call them or openly discuss my thoughts and feelings throughout the course of my entire case. Thus, my ongoing daily interactions with office staff, immediate and extended family members, and the various professionals who were involved in my defense were all sources of emotional, cognitive, behavioral, and interpersonal support and strength. These sources of healthy support, nurturance, and strength were constant deterrents to the manifestation of parataxic countertransference distortions and acting out on my part as I continued to see a very limited number of patients at this time. They were also deterrents to countertransference-related acting out in other areas of social functioning and interaction.

Finally, I continued both to discover and to relearn that my spirituality and basic faith in God were incredible sources of strength in this time of personal crisis. Prayer, meditation, spiritual introspection, and attending church on a near weekly basis became increasingly important in my life. The peace, tranquility, wisdom, and emotional comfort provided by Sunday Mass became a one-hour weekend experience that I found myself looking forward to—and I'm not a Catholic! The wisdom of forgiveness, letting go, praying for my enemies, kindness and love, living life one day at a time, acceptance, and many basic scripture stories and keys to living a more productive and meaningful life, as well as the

AA Big Book 12-step and other tools for living a sober and more sane life, all took on new relevance and meaning in my life. I found myself actually applying and attempting to live these principles in all my interactions with others on a daily basis. As a consequence of these realities, I began to experience and understand more fully the real inner strengths that I have possessed for years—perhaps forever—in the midst of one of the most turbulent and painful times in my life. I eventually discovered great personal strength at the core of my weakest and most vulnerable self—and God, spirituality, religion, and faith were at the core of this painful personal growth experience.

I was able to maintain my personal sanity, self-worth, and basic sense of professional competence and integrity throughout the course of this sixteen-month ordeal by consistently utilizing the various resources that have been briefly outlined in this epilogue. Most important and specifically related to the topic of this book, I was also able to use these tools and resources to minimize, resolve, and contain a plethora of countertransference reactions and dynamics that were related to the experience and process of being sued. In spite of the stress and emotional turmoil caused by this lawsuit, I was consistently able to utilize these cognitive, interpersonal, behavioral, physical, communicative, supportive, and spiritual resources to help me continue to help my clients. My personal feelings of hurt, distrust, anxiety, anger and rage, fear, and insecurity were not projected onto my clients and did not parataxically distort our psychotherapy relationships. I even continued to treat attorneys and their spouses and children and realized more clearly than ever that most attorneys are responsible, competent, and very decent human beings!

This major life experience simply reinforced a basic theme in this book—the ongoing and ever-changing life experiences of the counselor and psychotherapist continuously shape and affect the various countertransference-oriented parameters of the therapeutic relationship. Countertransference literally oozes from every pore and aspect of the counselor. Countertransference is ever-changing (Forrest, 2001) and an ever-present "red thread" that continuously impacts the therapeutic process and therapeutic alliance, and these realities will persist within the context of all counseling and therapeutic relationships in this new millennium.

Bibliography

Adams, D. B. (2000). Managing industrial injuries: Clinical objectivism and non-partisan practice. *Psychotherapy Bulletin, 35*(2), 20-24.

Aspy, D. N., Aspy, C. B., Russel, G., and Wedel, M. (2000). Carkhuff's human technology: A verification and extension of Kelly's (1977) suggestion to integrate the humanistic and technical components of counseling. *Journal of Counseling and Development, 78*(1), 29-37.

Beauchamp, T. L., and Childress, J. F. (1983). *Principles of biomedical ethics.* Oxford: Oxford University Press.

Bellack, A. S. (2000). Behavioral treatment for substance abuse in schizophrenia. *The Addictions Newsletter, 7*(2), 20-22.

Bleger, J. (1967). Psychoanalysis of the psychoanalytic frame. Internet. *Journal of Psychoanalysis,* 48:511-519.

Blum, H. (1987). Countertransference: Concepts and controversies. In E. Slakter (Ed.), *Countertransference* (pp. 87-104). Northvale, NJ: Jason Aronson, Inc.

Bratter, T. E. (1985). Special clinical psychotherapeutic concerns for alcoholic and drug-addicted individuals. In T. E. Bratter and G. G. Forrest (Eds.), *Alcoholism and substance abuse: Strategies for clinical intervention* (pp. 341-369). New York: Free Press.

Bratter, T. E. and Forrest, G. G. (Eds.) (1985). *Alcoholism and substance abuse: Strategies for clinical intervention.* New York: Free Press.

Brenner, C. (1977). *Psychoanalytic technique and psychic conflict.* New York: International Universities Press.

Britton, P. J., Cimini, K. T., and Rak, C. F. (1999). Techniques for teaching HIV counseling: An intensive experiential model. *Journal of Counseling and Development, 77*(2), 171-176.

Carruth, F. B. (2000). *The difficult client.* Paper presented at the Psychotherapy Associates, P.C., and co-sponsors, 26th Annual International "Addictive Disorders and Behavioral Health" Winter Symposium, January 27, Colorado Springs, CO.

Celenza, A. (1995). Love and hate in the countertransference supervisory concerns. *Psychotherapy: Theory, Research, Practice, and Training, 32*(2), 301-307.

Culbreth, J. R. and Borders, L. D. (1999). Perceptions of the supervisory relationship: Recovering and nonrecovering substance abuse counselors. *Journal of Counseling and Development, 77*(3), 330-338.

Curton, E. D. and Parker, B. (1998). *Implementing and managing dual-diagnosis programs.* Paper presented at the Psychotherapy Associates, P.C., 24th Annual International "Treatment of Addictive Disorders" Winter Symposium, January 26, Colorado Springs, CO.

Dalenberg, C. J. (2000). *Countertransference and the treatment of trauma.* Washington, DC: APA Books.

Deutsch, H. (1953/1926). Occult processes occurring during psychoanalysis. In G. Devereux (Ed.), *Psychoanalysis and the occult.* New York: International Universities Press.

Dove, W. R. (1995). Ethics training for the alcohol/drug abuse professional. *Alcohol Treatment Quarterly, 12*(4), 19-30.

Dove, W. R. (1997). *Ethics training.* Paper presented at the Psychotherapy Associates, P.C., 23rd Annual International "Treatment of Addictive Disorders" Winter Symposium, February 3, Colorado Springs, CO.

Emrick, C. D. (1979). Perspectives in clinical research: Relative effectiveness of alcohol abuse treatment. *Family and Community Health, 2*(2), 71-88.

Emrick, C. D. (1991). *The assessment and treatment of alcohol and drug problems: Special emphasis on community-based and self-help resources.* Paper presented at the Psychotherapy Associates, P.C., 17th Annual International "Treatment of Addictive Disorders" Winter Symposium, February 5, Colorado Springs, CO.

Fenichel, O. (1945). *The psychoanalytic theory of neurosis.* New York: W.W. Norton.

Ferenczi, S. (1950/1919). On the techniques of psychoanalysis. *Further contributions to the theory and technique of psycho-analysis* (pp. 177-189). London: Hogarth Press.

Fleiss, R. (1942). The metapsychology of the analyst. *Psychoanalytic Quarterly, 11,* 211-227.

Forrest, G. G. (1970). Transparency as a prognostic variable in psychotherapy. Unpublished doctoral dissertation. University of North Dakota, Grand Forks.

Forrest, G. G. (1978). *The diagnosis and treatment of alcoholism* (Second edition). Springfield, IL: Charles C Thomas.

Forrest, G. G. (1979). Setting alcoholics up for therapeutic failure. *Family and Community Health, 2*(2), 59-64.

Forrest, G. G. (1984). Psychotherapy of alcoholics and substance abusers: Outcome assessment revisited. *Family and Community Health, 2*(1), 40-50.

Forrest, G. G. (1985). Psychodynamically-oriented treatment of alcoholism and substance abuse. In T. E. Bratter and G. G. Forrest (Eds.), *Alcoholism and substance abuse: Strategies for clinical intervention* (pp. 220-245). New York: Free Press.

Forrest, G. G. (1991). Role slippage and adaptation in the alcoholic family system. *Family Dynamics of Addiction Quarterly, 1*(3), 315-339.

Forrest, G. G. (1992). *Confrontation in psychotherapy with the alcoholic.* Holmes Beach, FL: Learning Publications, Inc.

Forrest, G. G. (1994). *Alcoholism and human sexuality.* Northvale, NJ: Jason Aronson, Inc.

Forrest, G. G. (1996). *Chemical dependency and antisocial personality disorder: Psychotherapy and assessment strategies.* Binghamton, NY: The Haworth Press, Inc.

Forrest, G. G. (1997a). *Chemical dependency and mental health: Diagnosis and differential diagnosis.* Paper presented at the annual State Mental Health Association Conference, November 18, Bismarck, ND.

Forrest, G. G. (1997b). *Intensive psychotherapy of alcoholism.* Northvale, NJ: Jason Aronson, Inc.

Forrest, G. G. (1998a). *Countertransference in chemical dependency counseling.* Paper presented at the Psychotherapy Associates, P.C., 24th Annual International "Treatment of Addictive Disorders" Winter Symposium, January 27, Colorado Springs, CO.

Forrest, G. G. (1998b). *How to cope with a teenage drinker: Changing adolescent alcohol abuse.* Northvale, NJ: Jason Aronson, Inc.

Forrest, G. G. (1999). *Alcoholism, narcissism, psychopathology.* Northvale: Jason Aronson, Inc.

Forrest, G. G. (2000). The imprisoning of America. *Newsletter: International Academy of Behavioral Medicine, Counseling, and Psychotherapy, Inc., 20*(1) (Fall/Winter), 3.

Forrest, G. G. (2001). *How to live with a problem drinker.* Holmes Beach, FL: Learning Publications, Inc.

Forrest, G. G. and Gordon, R. (1990). *Substance abuse, homicide, and violent behavior.* New York: Gardner Press.

Freud, S. (1961/1910). Further prospects for psycho-analytic therapy. *The standard edition of the complete psychological works of Sigmund Freud* (Volume 11, pp. 141-142). London: Hogarth Press.

Freud, S. (1961/1912). Recommendations to physicians practicing psychoanalysis. *The standard edition of the complete psychological works of Sigmund Freud* (Volume 12, pp. 111-112).

Fromm-Reichmann, F. (1950). *Principles of intensive psychotherapy.* Chicago: University of Chicago Press.

Garrett, M. T. and Pichette, E. F. (2000). Red as an apple: Native American acculturation and counseling with or without reservation. *Journal of Counseling and Development, 78*(1), 3-13.

Gill, M. (1979). The analysis of the transference. *Journal of the American Psychoanalytic Association, 27*(Supplement), 263-288.

Giovacchini, P. (1979). Countertransference with primitive mental states. In L. Epstein and A. Feiner (Eds.), *Countertransference*. New York: Jason Aronson, Inc.

Gitelson, M. (1952). The emotional position of the analyst in the psychoanalytic situation. *International Journal of Psycho-Analysis, 33,* 1-10.

Glasser, W. (1965). *Reality therapy: A new approach to psychiatry.* New York: Harper and Row.

Glasser, W. (2000). *Reality therapy in action.* New York: HarperCollins Publishers, Inc.

Glover, E. (1927). Lectures on technique in psychoanalysis. *International Journal of Psycho-Analysis, 8,* 311-338.

Gorski, T. T. (1991). *Cocaine craving and relapse prevention.* Paper presented at the Psychotherapy Associates, P.C., 17th Annual International "Treatment of Addictive Disorders" Winter Symposium, February 26, Colorado Springs, CO.

Gorski, T. T. (1992). *Relapse prevention training.* Paper presented at the Psychotherapy Associates, P.C., 19th Annual International "Treatment of Addictive Disorders" Winter Symposium, February 7, Colorado Springs, CO.

Gorski, T. T. and Miller, M. (1986). *Staying sober: A guide for relapse prevention.* Independence, MO: Independence Press.

Greene, B. (1993). Psychotherapy with African American women: Integrating feminist and psychodynamic models. *Journal of Training and Practice in Professional Psychology, 7,* 49-66.

Greenson, R. (1971). The "real" relationship between the patient and the psychoanalyst. In M. Kanzer (Ed.), *The unconscious today* (pp. 213-232). New York: International Universities Press.

Hahn, W. K. (2000). Shame: Countertransference identifications in individual psycho-therapy. *Psychotherapy: Theory, research, practice, and training, 37*(1), 10-21.

Hansen, J. T. (2000). Psychoanalysis and humanism: A review and critical examination of integrationist efforts with some proposed resolutions. *Journal of Counseling and Development, 78*(1), 21-28.

Heil, S. H., Wong, C. J., and Higgins, S. T. (2000). Community reinforcement approach combined with contingent vouchers for the treatment of cocaine dependence. *The Addictions Newsletter, 7*(2), 9, 24-26.

Heimann, P. (1950). On countertransference. *International Journal of Psycho-Analysis, 31,* 81-84.

Helzer, J. E. and Pryzbeck, T. R. (1988). The co-occurrence of alcoholism and other psychiatric disorders in the general population and its impact on treatment. *Journal of Studies on Alcoholism, 49*(E), 219-224.

Hess, Allen K. (1980). *Psychotherapy supervision: Theory, research, and practice.* New York: John Wiley and Sons.

Hesselbrock, M. N., Meyer, R. E., and Kenner, J. J. (1985). Psycho-pathology in hospitalized alcoholics. *Archives in General Psychiatry, 42,* 1050-1055.

Hill, C. E. (2000). Training in helping skills. *Psychotherapy Bulletin, 35*(2), 39-41.

Hill, S. S. (1998). Multicultural mentoring initiative. *Psychotherapy Bulletin, 33*(1), 16-17.

Holt, J. L., Houg, B. L., and Romano, J. L. (2000). Spiritual wellness for clients with HIV/AIDS: Review of counseling issues. *Journal of Counseling and Development, 77*(2), 160-170.

Hountras, P. T. and Forrest, G. G. (1970). Personality characteristics and self-disclosure in a psychiatric outpatient population. *University of North Dakota College of Education Record, 55,* 206-213.

Howard, K. I. and Mahoney, M. T. (1996). How much outpatient therapy is enough? *Behavioral Healthcare Tomorrow, 5,* 44-50.

Irons, R. (1998). *Co-morbidity between domestic violence and addictive disease.* Paper presented at the Psychotherapy Associates, P.C., 24th Annual International "Treatment of Addictive Disorders" Winter Symposium, January 27, Colorado Springs, CO.

Irons, R. and Forrest, G. G. (1998). *Open forum: The vicissitudes of narcissism in addictions treatment.* Paper presented at the Psychotherapy Associates, P.C., 24th Annual International "Treatment of Addictive Disorders" Winter Symposium, January 28, Colorado Springs, CO.

Irons, R. and Schneider, J. P. (1999). *The wounded healer: Addiction-sensitive approach to the sexually exploitative professional.* Northvale, NJ: Jason Aronson, Inc.

Jourard, S. M. (1964). *The transparent self.* Princeton, NJ: Van Nostrand.

Kernberg, O. (1965). Notes on countertransference. *Journal of the American Psychoanalytic Association, 13,* 38-56.

Kernberg, O. (1975). *Borderline conditions and pathological narcissism.* Northvale, NJ: Jason Aronson, Inc.

Kitchener, K. S. (1986). Teaching applied ethics in counselor education: An integration of psychological processes and philosophical analysis. *Journal of Counseling and Development, 64,* 306-310.

Klauber, J. (1986). Elements of the psychoanalytic relationship and their therapeutic implications. In G. Konon (Ed.), *The British school of psy-*

choanalysis: The independent tradition (pp. 200-213). London: Free Association Books.

Knapp, S. and VandeCreek, L. (2000). Confidentiality under managed care: Ethical issues and recommendations. *Psychotherapy Bulletin, 35*(2), 25-32.

Knauert, A. P. (1979). The treatment of alcoholism in a community setting. *Family and Community Health, 2*(1), 91-102.

Knauert, A. P. (2000). *Advanced differential diagnosis of substance use disorders.* Paper presented at Psychotherapy Associates, P.C., and co-sponsors, 26th Annual International "Addictive Disorders and Behavioral Health" Winter Symposium, January 25, Colorado Springs, CO.

Kuhn, K. L. (1998). *Assessment and treatment of depression, affective disorders, and substance abuse.* Paper presented at the Psychotherapy Associates, P.C., 24th Annual International "Treatment of Addictive Disorders" Winter Symposium, January 27, Colorado Springs, CO.

La Roche, M. J. (1999). Culture, transference, and countertransference among Latinos. *Psychotherapy: Theory, Research, Practice and Training, 36*(4), 389-397.

Langs, R. (1978). *The listening process.* New York: Jason Aronson, Inc.

Lawson, G. and Lawson, A. (Eds.) (1992). *Adolescent substance abuse: Etiology, treatment and prevention.* Gaithersburg, MD: Aspen.

Levin, J. D. (1991). *Treatment of alcoholism and other addictions: A self-psychology approach.* Northvale, NJ: Jason Aronson, Inc.

Maroda, K. (1994). *The power of countertransference: Innovations in analytic technique.* Northvale, NJ: Jason Aronson, Inc.

Marotta, S. A. and Asner, K. K. (1999). Group psychotherapy for women with a history of incest: The research base. *Journal of Counseling and Development, 77*(3), 315-323.

McDougall, J. (1979). Primitive communication and the use of countertransference. In L. Epstein and A. Feiner (Eds.), *Countertransference* (pp. 267-303). New York: Jason Aronson, Inc.

Menninger, K. A. and Holzman, P. S. (1958). *Theory of psychoanalytic technique.* New York: Basic Books.

Nace, E. P. (1990). Subtance abuse and personality disorder. In P. F. O'Connel (Ed.), *Managing the dually-diagnosed patient: Current issues and clinical approaches.* Binghamton, NY: The Haworth Press, Inc.

Najavits, L. J., Griffin, M. L., Luborsky, L., Frank, A., Weiss, R. D., Liese, B. S., Thompson, H., Nakayama, E., Sigueland, C., Daley, D., and Onken, L. S. (1995). Therapists' emotional reactions to substance abusers: A new questionnaire and initial findings. *Psychotherapy: Theory, Research, Practice, and Training, 32*(4), 669-677.

Neumann, D. A. and Gamble, S. J. (1995). Issues in professional development of psychotherapists: Countertransference and vicarious traumatization in the new trauma therapist. *Psychotherapy: Theory, Research, Practice, and Training, 32*(2), 341-347.

Okonji, J. M. A. (1998). *Managing diversity in the workplace.* Paper presented at the Psychotherapy Associates, P.C., 24th Annual International "Treatment of Addictive Disorders" Winter Symposium, January 27, Colorado Springs, CO.

Okonji, J. M. A., Ososki, J. N., and Pulos, S. (1998). Preferred style and ethnicity of counselors by African American males. *Journal of Black Psychology, 22*(3), 329-339.

Pattison, E. M. (1987). *Borderline, narcissistic, and addictive disorders: Differential diagnosis and treatment considerations.* Paper presented at the Psychotherapy Associates, P.C., 13th Annual International "Treatment of Addictive Disorders" Winter Symposium, February 2, Colorado Springs, CO.

Peterson, S. (2000). Multicultural perspective on middle-class women's identity development. *Journal of Counseling and Development, 78*(1), 63-71.

Pope, K. (1986). How clients are harmed by sexual contact with mental health professionals: The syndrome and its prevalence. *Journal of Counseling and Development, 65,* 222-226.

Pope, K. (1991). Dual relations in psychotherapy. *Ethics and Behavior, 1,* 21-34.

Reich, W. (1945/1933). *Character analysis: Principles and techniques for psychoanalysts in practice and training* (Second edition). New York: Orgone Institute.

Reik, T. (1948). *Listening with the third ear.* New York: Farrar, Strauss, and Young.

Rounsaville, B. J., Eyre, S. L., Weissman, M. M., and Kleber, H. D. (1983). The antisocial opiate addict. *Advances in Alcohol and Substance Abuse, 2*(4), 29-42.

Savage, C. (1987). Countertransference in the therapy of schizophrenics. In E. Slakter (Ed.), *Countertransference* (pp. 115-130). Northvale, NJ: Jason Aronson, Inc.

Schultz, R. E. and Hughes, C. G. (1995). Countertransference in the treatment of pathological narcissism. *Psychotherapy: Theory, Research, Practice, and Training, 32*(4), 601-607.

Searles, H. (1958). The schizophrenic's vulnerability to the therapist's unconscious processes. *Journal of Nervous and Mental Disease, 127,* 247-262.

Searles, H. (1965). *Collected papers on schizophrenia and related subjects.* London: Horgarth; New York: International Universities Press.

Searles, H. (1975). The patient as therapist to his analyst. In P. Giovacchini (Ed.), *Tactics and techniques in psychoanalytic therapy:* Volume 2, *Countertransference* (pp. 95-151). New York: Jason Aronson, Inc.

Searles, H. F. (1987). Countertransference as a path to understanding and helping the patient. In E. Slakter (Ed.), *Countertransference* (pp. 131-163). Northvale, NJ: Jason Aronson, Inc.

Sena, D. A. (1993). *Neuropsychological factors in the assessment and treatment of substance use disorders.* Paper presented at the Psychotherapy Associates, P.C., 19th Annual International "Treatment of Addictive Disorders" Winter Symposium, February 7, Colorado Springs, CO.

Shaffer, H. J. (1994). Denial, ambivalence, and countertransferential hate. In. J. D. Levin and R. H. Weiss (Eds.), *The dynamics and treatment of alcoholism: Essential papers* (pp. 421-437). Northvale, NJ: Jason Aronson, Inc.

Slakter, E. (1987). Reality issues and countertransference. In E. Slakter (Ed.), *Countertransference* (pp. 219-226). Northvale, NJ: Jason Aronson, Inc.

Stekel, W. (1929). *Sadism and masochism:* Volume 1. London: Liveright Publishing Co.

Stern, A. (1924). On the countertransference in psychoanalysis. *Psychoanalytic Review, 2,* 166-174.

Strupp, H. H. (1997). Research, practice, and managed care. *Psychotherapy: Theory, Research, Practice, and Training, 34*(1), 91-94.

Stucky, J. (1995). *Treatment of sexual compulsions.* Paper presented at the Psychotherapy Associates, P.C., 21st Annual International "Treatment of Addictive Disorders" Winter Symposium, February 5, Colorado Springs, CO.

Sullivan, H. S. (1953). *The interpersonal theory of psychiatry.* New York: Norton.

Tansey, M. J. and Burke, W. F. (1989). *Understanding counter-transference: From projective identification to empathy.* Hillsdale, NJ: The Analytic Press.

Terrell, F. and Terrell, S. (1984). Race of counselor, client, sex, cultural mistrust level, and premature termination from counseling among black clients. *Journal of Counseling Psychology, 31,* 371-375.

Thompson, C. E., Worthington, R., and Atkinson, D. R. (1994). Counselor content orientation, counselor race, and black women's cultural mistrust level and self-disclosure. *Journal of Counseling Psychology, 41,* 155-161.

Tower, L. (1956). Countertransference. *Journal of the American Psychoanalytic Association, 4,* 224-255.

Truax, C. B. and Carkhuff, R. R. (1967). *Toward effective counseling and psychotherapy.* Chicago: Aldine.

Utsey, S. O., Ponterotto, J. G., Reynolds, A. L., and Cancelli, A. A. (2000). Racial discrimination, coping, life satisfaction, and self-esteem among African Americans. *Journal of Counseling and Development, 78*(1), 72-80.

Wallace, J. (1985). *Alcoholism: New light on the disease.* Newport, RI: Edgehill Publications.

Walsh, W. F. (1998). The crisis in confidentiality in the setting of managed care. *The Independent Practitioner, 18*(1), 25-28.

Wegscheider, S. (1981). *Another chance: Hope and health for the alcoholic family.* Palo Alto, CA: Science and Behavior Books, Inc.

Weiss, Ronna H. (1994). Countertransference issues in treating the alcoholic patient: Institutional and clinical reactions. In J. D. Levin and R. H. Weiss (Eds.), *The dynamics and treatment of alcoholism: Essential papers.* Northvale, NJ: Jason Aronson, Inc.

Wilsnack, S. C. and Beckman, L. J. (1984). *Alcohol problems in women.* New York: The Guilford Press.

Wilsnack, S. C. and Klassen, A. (1988). *Sexuality, sexual dysfunction, and women's drinking.* Paper presented at the Psychotherapy Associates, P.C., 14th Annual International "Treatment of Addictive Disorders" Winter Symposium, February 4, Colorado Springs, CO.

Winnicott, D. (1949). Hate in the countertransference. *International Journal of Psycho-Analysis, 30,* 69-74.

Zimberg, S. (1982). *The clinical management of alcoholism.* New York, Brunner/Mazel, Inc.

Index

Page numbers followed by the letter "t" indicate tables.

Order Your Own Copy of
This Important Book for Your Personal Library!

COUNTERTRANSFERENCE IN CHEMICAL DEPENDENCY COUNSELING

_____in hardbound at $34.95 (ISBN: 0-7890-1523-4)

_____in softbound at $19.95 (ISBN: 0-7890-1524-2)

COST OF BOOKS_____

OUTSIDE USA/CANADA/
MEXICO: ADD 20%_____

POSTAGE & HANDLING_____
(US: $4.00 for first book & $1.50
for each additional book)
Outside US: $5.00 for first book
& $2.00 for each additional book)

SUBTOTAL_____

in Canada: add 7% GST_____

STATE TAX_____
(NY, OH & MIN residents, please
add appropriate local sales tax)

FINAL TOTAL_____
(If paying in Canadian funds,
convert using the current
exchange rate, UNESCO
coupons welcome.)

❑ **BILL ME LATER:** ($5 service charge will be added)
(Bill-me option is good on US/Canada/Mexico orders only;
not good to jobbers, wholesalers, or subscription agencies.)

❑ Check here if billing address is different from
shipping address and attach purchase order and
billing address information.

Signature_____

❑ **PAYMENT ENCLOSED: $_____**

❑ **PLEASE CHARGE TO MY CREDIT CARD.**

❑ Visa   ❑ MasterCard   ❑ AmEx   ❑ Discover
❑ Diner's Club   ❑ Eurocard   ❑ JCB

Account # _____

Exp. Date_____

Signature_____

Prices in US dollars and subject to change without notice.

NAME_____

INSTITUTION_____

ADDRESS_____

CITY_____

STATE/ZIP_____

COUNTRY_____ COUNTY (NY residents only)_____

TEL_____ FAX_____

E-MAIL_____

May we use your e-mail address for confirmations and other types of information? ❑ Yes ❑ No
We appreciate receiving your e-mail address and fax number. Haworth would like to e-mail or fax special
discount offers to you, as a preferred customer. **We will never share, rent, or exchange your e-mail address
or fax number.** We regard such actions as an invasion of your privacy.

Order From Your Local Bookstore or Directly From
The Haworth Press, Inc.
10 Alice Street, Binghamton, New York 13904-1580 • USA
TELEPHONE: 1-800-HAWORTH (1-800-429-6784) / Outside US/Canada: (607) 722-5857
FAX: 1-800-895-0582 / Outside US/Canada: (607) 722-6362
E-mail: getinfo@haworthpressinc.com
PLEASE PHOTOCOPY THIS FORM FOR YOUR PERSONAL USE.
www.HaworthPress.com

BOF00